A CUP OF COFFEE WITH "MY" DENTIST

10 OF AMERICA'S LEADING DENTISTS SHARE THEIR STORIES, EXPERIENCES, AND INSIGHTS

Kathy Jacobsen, D.M.D.
Randy Van Ittersum

TRADEMARKS

Zoom!® is a registered trademark of Discus Dental, Inc. Sinsational Smile® is a registered trademark of Sinsational Smile, Inc. Invisalign® is a registered trademark of Align Technology, Inc. BOTOX® is a registered trademark of Allergan, Inc. Motrin® is a registered trademark of McNEIL-PPC, Inc. Crest® is a registered trademark of the Proctor & Gamble Company. VELscope® is a registered trademark of LED Medical Diagnostics, Inc. e.max ® is a registered trademark of Ivoclar Vivadent. LipStaT™ is a registered trademark of the Dr. Monish Bhola. All other trademarks are the property of their respective owners and/or their affiliates in the United States or other countries, and may not be used without written permission. The use of these trademarks within this publication were not authorized by, nor is this publication sponsored by or associated with, the trademark owners. Rutherford Publishing House is not associated with any product or vendor mentioned in this book.

Rutherford Publishing House
PO Box 969
Ramseur, NC 27316
www.RutherfordPublishingHouse.com

Cover photo: ardni/Bigstock.com
Book layout/design: Richard E. Spalding

ISBN-10: 0692520716
ISBN-13: 978-0692520710

Legal Disclaimer

The content of this book should be used for informational purposes only. It does not create any doctor-patient relationship with any reader and should not be construed as medical advice. If you need medical advice, please contact a doctor in your community who can assess the specifics of your situation.

Every effort has been made to make this book as complete and as accurate as possible, but no warranty is implied. The information provided is on an "as is" basis. The publisher shall have neither liability nor responsibility to any person or entity with respect to any loss or damages arising from the information contained in this book.

TABLE OF CONTENTS

Acknowledgements

We all want to thank our husbands and wives, fathers and mothers, and everybody who has played a role in shaping our lives and our attitudes.

To all the clients we've had the honor of working with, who shaped our understanding of the difficulty of this time for you and your families. It has been our privilege to serve each and every one of you.

INTRODUCTION

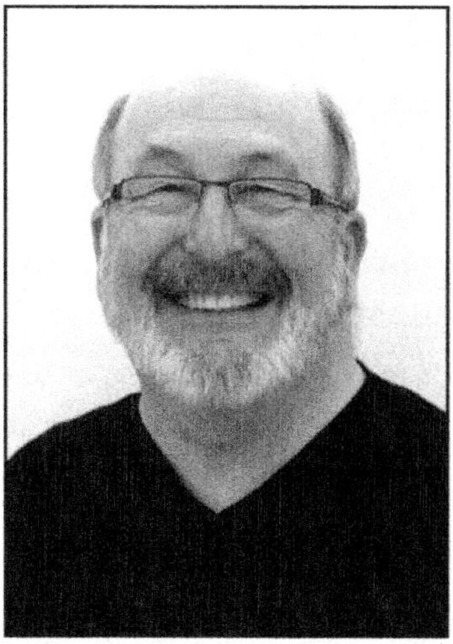

Contributing Author:
Randy Van Ittersum
Host & Founder – Business Leader Spotlight Show

Dentist get a bad rap. Even though the dentist is often the first responder in the battle for a patient's healthy body, we sometimes fall prey to the fear that continues to circulate around this group of professionals sparked by long-ago stories about bad dental chair experiences. This book, *A Cup of Coffee with My Dentist*, hopes to change that—at least for a few dentists, anyway.

This book is meant to take the place of, or at least augment, that initial chat you might have enjoyed with your dentist, had your mouth not been full of his fingers at the time. (Remarkably, they seem to understand what you say with your mouth numb and sprouting instruments. We suppose it's a course requirement in Dental school.) Our goal is for you to get to know your "physician of the mouth" a little better. Think of this book as an introduction.

Here, you will be introduced to some of the dedicated individuals who devote their days to caring for your mouth and, in so doing, make the rest of your body function the way it was meant to. You'll learn about their backgrounds, what inspires them, the fuel that drives them, and the reasons that drive seems unquenchable.

Some of the practitioners whom we've selected for this publication have stories of childhoods spent in other nations and the challenges that came with assimilating into American culture. One young girl came alone to the United States from Taiwan, leaving her family and home behind her in pursuit of her highest potential. She still seeks that potential every day.

You'll hear stories of unrelenting parents whose emphasis on education and excellence molded young students into gifted professionals whose commitment to the health and well being of their patients may already be an inspiration within your own community. These dentists are steeped in the need to aspire to the top in everything they do. With them, mediocrity isn't an option.

One common theme emerges as one turns these pages. Each of these professionals talks about the "family feeling" they nurture within their offices. They all seem patiently yet doggedly determined to erase your "bad dentist" experiences and replace them with trust and confidence. Understanding, as they do, that trust is not easily won and can easily be forfeited, these dentists go to astonishing lengths to make and keep you comfortable during your visits to them. More importantly, they are fostering generations of youngsters who simply have never had bad experiences in the dental chair. These kids have the edge of early acclimation to the dentist's office followed by regular checkups that serve to nip problems like decay in the bud. Early diagnosis and treatment ultimately lead to less dental intervention and, of course, no pain. Of special interest to parents: with checkups early and often, there are far fewer bills for extensive repairs, root canals, or expensive treatment of gum disease.

The dentists whose stories reside within the covers of this book want you to know and understand them better as human beings and, as a bonus, they will teach you more about your teeth than you ever knew was possible.

- When should your child see his dentist for the first time?
- What is "sedation dentistry," and are you a candidate?
- When the baby's pacifier MUST go.
- Why not just pull that broken molar? Do you really need it?
- Are dental implants right for you?
- How long should I expect my natural teeth to last? (Can you spell f-o-r-e-v-e-r?)

Some of the biggest light-bulb moments come during the discussions around preventative dentistry. Here's just one sample bombshell.

Q: Is a pint of apple juice every day enough for my 2-year-old?

A: EGAD! Sugary drinks like apple juice, canned soda, chocolate milk, and those handy little juice boxes *have no place in a child's daily diet*. One such drink on a single, special day each week is more than enough! (Who knew?)

And just wait until you hear about that bedtime bottle of milk your toddler expects each night.

You will be interested in learning that early checkups and intervention can prevent the need for expensive orthodontic work in the teenage years. (And we mean really early.) Proper alignment of teeth and, yes, even jaws, takes place very early in the bone-growing process. Those parents who wait until all of the precious little baby teeth fully emerge may be sealing the orthodontic fate of their children. Not only can jaw problems be identified early, so can many other systemic issues.

The same plaque we encourage our little ones to remove twice daily with the trusty toothbrush can, if left untended, travel throughout the body to wreak havoc elsewhere. And, should decay and infection become a problem in the mouth, you may trust that those germs are invading other tissues. Early training in oral hygiene is one very good way to ensure overall body health. The good men and women who share their stories here don't equivocate about the value of preventative dental care. It seems they build entire careers around the concept.

A Cup of Coffee with My Dentist also provides unexpected insights through the work of two dentists in New Jersey. These dentists work within underserved urban areas with goals that include much more than healthy teeth. Through an ambitious educational program that begins with day-care and follows children through high school, these doctors are helping immigrant parents understand that "old world ways" are not always the best ways. They demonstrate that among the opportunities available on American soil are the benefits—physical and emotional— of owning a big, healthy smile. Such smiles can be keys that open doors to prosperity later in life. (Studies tell us that other people think a person with a healthy-looking smile is probably smarter than those who have a less sterling grin.)

Certainly the smile factor extends to grown-up patients as well. The dentists whose stories fill these pages share a common concern for people whose dental care history—or lack thereof— has left them with missing or damaged teeth. People in these circumstances go to sad lengths to hide their imperfections. From growing a moustache to fingertips that invariably cover the mouth when it opens to speak or to laugh, people develop elaborate disguises, most of which only end up calling attention to the problem. Not only can dental "blemishes" do insurmountable damage to fragile self-esteem, but they can also pinion capable people in miserable circumstances in both their personal and professional lives.

People with missing, stained, or crooked teeth have real handicaps in the world of employment and industry, and it's an unnecessary burden for them to bear. Smiles can be restored and health can be improved by dental intervention, the cost of which can be "handled" through insurance policies, payment arrangements, or even credit cards. These dentists recognize that the cost for their services can be a difficult weight to carry, but because there are critical reasons to have the work done, these professionals are prepared to point the way to some of the creative financing options available out there.

In short, *A Cup of Coffee with My Dentist* is a personal book. It is written from the hearts of men and women who take their calling very, very seriously for very personal reasons. Those reasons include you, your family, and even your community as a whole. Please accept this invitation to get to know the person in the white lab coat.

Randy Van Ittersum
Host & Founder – Business Leader Spotlight Show

1

The Rewards Of Being A Dentist In An Intimate Dental Practice

by Kathy Jacobsen, D.M.D.

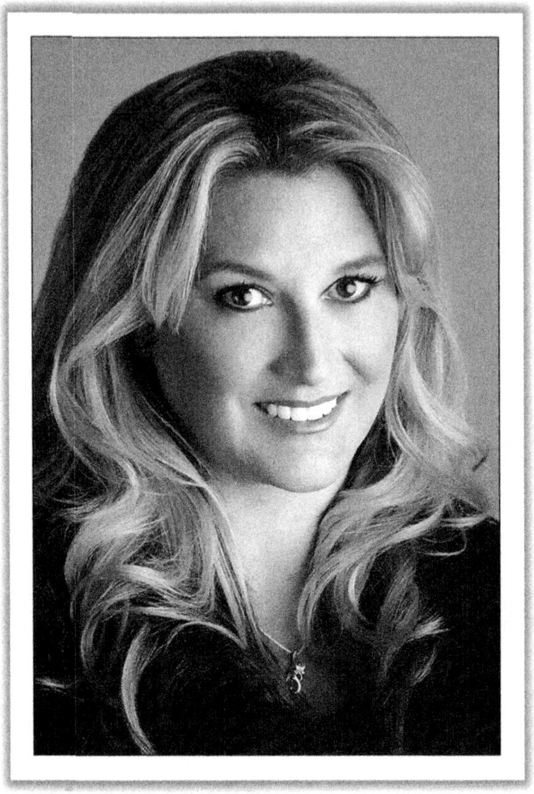

Kathy Jacobsen, D.M.D.

Contemporary Dentistry
Gilbert, Arizona
www.azdentistry.com

Dr. Kathy Jacobsen earned her DMD degree in 1994 from the University Medical and Dental School of New Jersey. Since then, her contagious enthusiasm has allowed her to build a thriving practice focusing on adult restorative and cosmetic dentistry, and general family dentistry. From the beginning of her career, Dr. Jacobsen has been dedicated to building long-term patient relationships and staying abreast of the latest advancements in the field of dental science. She continually expands her skills and knowledge through constant continuing education courses, including the Las Vegas Institute to study advanced dental anterior esthetics. Her team accompanies her for additional training in their areas of expertise. Dr. Jacobsen is a member of the American Dental Association, Arizona Dental Association, Academy of General Dentists, American Association of Women Dentists and the American Academy of Cosmetic Dentists. She is the mother of three, a boy and two girls, and is a strong believer in giving back to the community. Each year she and her staff hold a community dental day where they treat local kids free of charge. Involved in Smiles for Life, as a Crown Council dentist, Dr. Jacobsen donates proceeds from teeth whitening to seriously ill, disabled, and underprivileged children in the Phoenix area. She is also associated with the Teammates for Kids Foundation, which contributes financial resources to selected nonprofit organizations that effectively serve and benefit children with an emphasis on health, education and inner city services. In addition to all of this, Dr. Jacobsen donates to local animal shelters and to our troops who are serving our country.

Dr. Jacobsen is highly trained in the art and science of creating happy, healthy smiles through professional restorative and cosmetic dentistry. Contemporary Dentistry, in Gilbert, is here to help you obtain and maintain strong, healthy teeth and a beautiful smile. We designed our entire practice around providing state-of-the-art dental care in a comfortable, family friendly environment. We will make your dental experience sensational!

Our entire staff is dedicated to continuous improvement and constantly attends many professional seminars and education courses to stay at the very top of our areas of expertise. We look forward to meeting you in person!

The Rewards Of Being A Dentist In An Intimate Dental Practice

How I Became A Dentist And The Greatest Influences In My Life

I am a transplant to Arizona. I grew up on the East Coast in New Jersey as one of three children; I have one brother and one sister. Living so close to New York City, I had access to everything the Big Apple has to offer, including some of the world's best museums and theaters. My dentist was a big influence in helping me choose a career. I always had a love for science, and he told me that dentistry might be a good career choice for me. He invited me into his office so that I could get a behind-the-scenes look at the world of dentistry and I was "hooked."

I began dental school at Fairleigh Dickinson, which closed while I was in the process of receiving my degree. I then transferred to South Carolina, but I wasn't a southern girl, so I transferred back to New Jersey and graduated from the University of Medicine and Dentistry of New Jersey. I then decided to move to Arizona to start my dental practice. My family and I have lived in Arizona for 18 years. I am married with three children: a 19-year-old, a 14-year-old, and an 8-year-old. Skylar, Calla, and Casey take up all of my time away from the practice. I also have two stepsons and three step-grandchildren. I am a busy mom and a busy dentist.

I love being in Arizona. The state has a lot to offer. Arizona is really growing. I think our community in Gilbert has been one of the fastest-growing communities in the country for several years in a row. It has been a great place to start my practice. Gilbert and Las Vegas were two of the fastest-growing areas in the country for several years. The population in Gilbert increased from 30,000 to 200,000 in a very short time. When I came, there were not as many dentists as there are today. There's been a recent influx of dentists because of the two dental schools in Arizona that were opened after I moved here. I am happy with my practice, and I am happy with how my practice has grown. I am proud to have served Gilbert for almost twenty years.

My practice is a small dental family. Two hygienists work with me on a daily basis. I have an associate who does all of our oral surgery and implant placement. I am considering bringing on board an endodontist for our patients who prefer having treatment at my office. I do not want to grow my practice too much more beyond a small family practice because it works perfectly. In the past, I did grow my practice larger, but I decided to return to a smaller, more intimate practice. I like it exactly where it is right now.

The two most important things that have influenced my daily life as an adult are my family and my patients. If I am not working, I am spending time with my kids. My daughter is an active equestrian and my son is working on his black belt in karate. We love to travel as well as do things locally. We are definitely animal lovers with dogs, cats, a horse, and guinea pigs.

I consider my patients to be part of the family as well. I love my patients' stories. I love them being part of our dental family. That makes our practice different from some other dental practices. My patients have my cell phone number and they know they can text me. I am there if they need me. Some dentists have told me, "You don't want your patients on your Facebook page. You don't want your patients to know where you live." I prefer to practice differently. I know patients feel very comfortable with me. Patients like the friendly atmosphere of my practice. They prefer not being a chart or a number. My patients are friends on my Facebook page. They like seeing the pictures of my kids, and I enjoy seeing the pictures of their families as well.

My basic dental philosophy is to treat my patients like my family. I give them the options that I would offer to my own family, and I tell them what I would do if I were in their situation. Our practice is a little different. Most patients come into our office and say, "It's so different. It feels like we're part of the family." I have personally visited other places, and it does not feel like you are a part of the family. My patients enjoy feeling like they belong. They know that I am honest with them and I am not trying to sell them anything that they do not truly need. They know that I am doing what is necessary because I care about them.

They sense that I am genuine. You do not need to talk about integrity when you are honest because people will know that you are honest by the way you act, not by what you profess. I hate the new catchphrase "integrity," because when someone talks about "integrity," that person usually does not have it within himself. I think that people know if you care or if you are simply trying to make a sale. I treat my patients the way that I want to be treated. We have events during the year to show our patients how much we appreciate them. As far as dentistry goes, our philosophy is conservative. We want to save as much of the tooth structure as possible because that is what we would want to do if it was our own teeth.

The Future Of Dentistry

Dentistry has really changed since I graduated. Large group practices are replacing the single doctor practices. Corporate dental offices are starting to come into town, and I am not sure that they provide the care or concern that a patient needs. I believe they are more concerned with the bottom line—that they have a bigger focus on dental management and profit rather than patient care. If you are focusing on production and numbers, you lose something in the care. I think that this is the direction these corporate practices are moving toward. My new assistants who have worked in corporate dental offices and patients who have gone to corporate offices say it is so different from our practice. A different dentist treats the patient with a different philosophy every time that the patient comes into the office. I do not think that the corporate dental concept is a good thing for the public. I believe patients prefer smaller dentist-owned and operated practices where the patients and their needs are the primary focus.

Dental technology is also changing every day with new techniques and new products. Everything is getting easier and better for the patients. Dental materials have become better and better. Crowns and veneers today look very much like natural teeth. They have translucency and vitality that was just not present a few years ago. Invisible braces can be worn to straighten teeth. Implants can replace a broken tooth. I love that we no longer need to perform a heroic effort to save a tooth because now our implant procedures have a very high success rate. When I was first out of school, we would bisect the tooth to perform a root canal to save half of the tooth. Now we take out the tooth and replace it with an implant for a long-term solution that is more predictable. Smile makeovers produce life-changing results. Television shows have allowed the public to see some of the options available. Patients are happy with the ease in which they can enhance their appearance. A dazzling smile is now an affordable reality.

Your smile is the first thing people notice about you. Ninety-six percent of the population believes that a good smile is important.

People often don't understand that they lose some of their self-esteem when they lose a tooth or multiple teeth. The embarrassment translates into a loss of self-confidence. Patients will stay away from the dentist for years and the teeth will be neglected. It takes a lot for a patient to come in after a long absence and seek treatment. I welcome them and say, "Let's fix it. We can't go back in time, but let's take it from this point and give you back what you had or give you something better." I love that we can replace teeth with implants for a long-term solution. Implants have been used since the 1970s. The implant will feel like one of your own teeth; you can chew as if it were one your own teeth, and even multiple implants will look great. As the population ages, people want to maintain their natural teeth. They no longer want to wear dentures like Grandma used to wear. They will want to have their teeth back. If they lose a tooth, they will replace it with an implant to have their teeth for the rest of their life instead of going the dentures route.

Digital technology is wonderful. Digital x-rays have less radiation exposure for patients. Digital impressions allow for an easy way to transfer information to the lab which fabricates our restorations. We do not need take messy impressions anymore. We can take a digital image, send it over to the lab, and they can fabricate the tooth. Intraoral cameras allow patients to see what we see. There have been so many advances that benefit both dentist and patient.

Personal Healthcare And Dental Care

I hoped to see a change with dental care included in the new healthcare plans, but that has not really happened. The new plans under the Affordable Healthcare Act have not been very inclusive. Some of our patients do have good dental care plans;

but so many people are only covered minimally or not at all. Americans want dental insurance to cover everything and are very disappointed when they find out the coverage limits may only be for one thousand dollars. People really need to make the connection between dental health and overall health. Patients can't truly be healthy with existing dental problems. With all of the changes that are occurring in healthcare, perhaps changes can be made to include the mouth as part of the whole body that needs treatment. I do not like the separation between medical issues and dental ones, because the body doesn't really differentiate. If a person is going to be healthy, the whole body must be healthy. Dental problems are very common. In our charitable work, we see children with severe dental issues. Kids are missing days of school because they have toothaches and dental infections which are going untreated. These kids have problems that are not being addressed. Insurance coverage will certainly help with access to care for more individuals and families, but dental insurance needs to keep up and cover at least the basic.

Being Afraid Of The Dentist

It's said that half of the population does not go to the dentist because of fear. I would like to let patients know that there are many different ways to make your visit comfortable. If you have some anxiety, nitrous oxide or laughing gas is wonderful. Medication helps patients feel less fearful about having a dental procedure. In our office we use oral triazolam to sedate some patients. The pill puts patients in a twilight sleep so they are still able to respond.

We also offer IV sedation for dental-phobics who are so fearful that they cannot be awake during the procedure. There are risks involved with general anesthesia, so we reserve this for the most fearful of patients. Some of my patients were so anxious that they could not even have an X-ray taken without some type of medication. With IV sedation, the patient goes to sleep. When the patient wakes up, the dental procedure is over. There is also an amnesiac effect, so they do not remember the procedure at all. The experience is pleasant.

Many patients have had a terrible experience in the past and won't visit a dentist unless it is an absolute emergency. Our office likes to educate patients on the different levels of sedation that are used to make patients comfortable. Our team stresses the importance of having a pleasant experience in the office. Patient comfort is our top priority. We even offer those same options for patients who are simply having their teeth cleaned or only having X-rays, because everyone's fear is different and everyone's fear is real. When patients are informed of the options, they let friends and relatives know and we are able to treat many who would otherwise not come to the dentist at all.

Fearful and anxious patients need to be introduced to dentistry again slowly. They need to feel comfortable with the practice and the doctor. Sometimes they need to come into the office for an interview with us so they can see our office and chat a little bit to feel more comfortable. With a new dentist, patients may feel unsure and unfamiliar with the dentist or the staff, so we refer them to our website to get an overview of the facility and team. New patients can come in, meet me and the team, and see the office so they can feel a level of comfort before they come in for dental work. I strive to make the new patients feel welcome and listened to. We have had much success using this process with our new patients, especially the fearful ones who haven't been to the dentist in 10 to 20 years.

Dealing With Dental Emergencies

Our office is different in the way that we handle dental emergencies. We have the patients call or text me directly and I get right back to them. In five minutes, I can jump in the car and run down to the office. My patients know that I am always available and that makes them feel comfortable. They like having the ability to text me with a question or call if they have a concern. Regardless of the emergency, from a broken filling to an avulsed tooth, they know that I am there for them and I know that they appreciate that.

Patients don't receive this level of care in a corporate setting. Someone answers the phone and takes a message whether it's an emergency or not. Then they refer it to whoever is on call to call in a prescription; they do not really seem to care that much. Some patients have told me that they have a dental plan and must go to a certain dental practice, but no one will answer their phone calls when there is an emergency. Of course, I will come right in for them, but you will not get that in a corporate setting. It has not been my experience and it has not been my patients' experience, either.

What Is Cosmetic Dentistry?

I think cosmetic dentistry is any dental work that makes someone look good and feel better. Many people believe that cosmetic dentistry must be extensive, with the patient's mouth full of veneers or crowns. However, we can fix one tooth and change the patient's smile and boost his or her self-esteem. First impressions are very important; your smile is a large part of the impression you make when meeting someone. Cosmetic dentistry can be as simple as teeth whitening to brighten your smile, replacing a missing tooth, or adding veneers. An attractive smile is important to all aspects of life, from your love life to your business life. We love what we can do for people through cosmetic dentistry.

Enhancing the smile can change someone's life. Confidence is boosted. After doing many smile makeovers, I have never had anyone say, "I wish I never did it." Almost everyone says, "Why did I wait so long?" People often don't realize the impact of their smile on their life until they change it. Generally, smile makeovers are not uncomfortable. With so many financing options, it is now an affordable way for people to change something about themselves that could be holding them back from living a fuller life.

In several smile makeover contests, individuals submitted a story telling why they needed a smile makeover. The first time, we had to pick three winners because we could not narrow down our choices to just one. One winner was a girl who did not want to leave her house because her teeth were so bad. She was not functioning in society, did not have any money, and had been in an abusive relationship. Our smile makeover changed her entire life—we redid the whole smile, not just veneers. She went out to meet people. She got a job. She lost weight. She found a new spouse. I do not know if all of that was due to her teeth, but the fact that she did not leave the house until her teeth were fixed meant that the smile makeover was at least partly responsible for the dramatic change in her life.

Every day, I do fillings and crowns, and I enable people to have teeth that function and do not hurt. Changing someone's life is the part that I like the best. One gentleman got a smile makeover and he is now a totally different person. His wife said he was always a friendly man, but he had a big, long mustache that partially hid his smile. When we finished the smile makeover, he trimmed his mustache to show off his smile.

People find ways to compensate for their teeth not being the way they want. Men cover their mouth when laughing. Women don't smile. It's important to be able to smile. I feel badly for people who don't smile because they feel ashamed of their teeth. I did not have very pretty teeth in my growing-up years. As a teenager, I had my teeth bonded. It made such a difference in my self-esteem. Over the years, I have had my teeth redone into a beautiful smile. People who have smile makeovers come back and tell us, "I'm always smiling now. I am so happy." Some patients who have had smile makeovers later tell us, "People used to think I was always mad. I wasn't mad, but I didn't smile. Now everybody thinks I'm always happy because I'm always smiling."

You are more approachable when you are smiling. You are perceived as more friendly. Studies say you are even perceived as more intelligent if you smile. I believe that a good smile is important for people, a way for them to express themselves. So many people get to the point of their teeth breaking down so they do not go out and they do not smile. There are so many options today to improve the way we look and feel about ourselves. Helping patients achieve the smile they have always dreamed of is affordable and within reach. My favorite part of dentistry is doing just that. It is very rewarding to see patients' responses when they see their new look.

The Process Of Cosmetic Dentistry

Everybody has different options for cosmetic dentistry. Some people only need teeth whitening or some gingival recontouring. Some need braces or extensive rehabilitation. It is important for patients to come into the office for a consultation so that we can learn what they want and discuss all of their options. I think everyone should know what services are available to them. A patient can be ready for a change or they may wait a year before coming back to schedule the work. They may have to get their finances in order or get their mindset ready to make a change. Some people take a few years and some people do it the next day. In either case, we discuss all of the options for developing a good game plan for them when they are ready to begin.

We give the patient a list of options (single-tooth implants, bridges, partial dentures, crowns, veneers, etc.), and then discuss the pros and cons of each option with the patient, as well as the costs and any risks. We also discuss "no replacement" as the last option. We base the care plan on what the patient needs, from a single tooth to a full mouth reconstruction. Listening to the patients' desires helps to form a treatment plan that is what they really want. Patients have been looking at themselves in the mirror, they know what they want to change and what they have come to love about their smile.

Implant Dentistry: Options To Replace Missing Teeth

If we are trying to save a questionable tooth by heroic means, we do a root canal. We build up the tooth and put a crown on it. The patient spends a lot of money and we do a lot of work for a tooth that may last two years. At that point, it is better to say, "This tooth will last you a few years if we do all of this, or we can remove the tooth and put in an implant that will last for many years." Many times, patients want long-term solutions, so I tell them, "If you have money and you want to spend all of this time to save this tooth for two or three years, that's certainly your prerogative. If it were my mouth, I'd probably take it out and have the implant placed. That way, I'd have something that's going to last, and I'm spending my money once instead of spending my money twice."

Many patients decide to have the implant rather than the root canal. In most cases, we remove the tooth and put in a bone graft at the same time. We then place the implant in the bone graft and allow it to heal. After looking at a broken-down, painful tooth, we say, "We can get rid of this tooth and place the implant at the same time—in one visit." It heals for a few months and then we restore it at that time. It is certainly a better method of treatment than trying to save the tooth at all costs. That is what we did in dentistry when I first graduated from dental school: saving the tooth and charging the patient $3,000 for something that only lasted for two years. Sometimes I think we wasted their money, but implants were not very good 25 years ago, and the success rate was not as high. Now dentistry has evolved.

A Healthy Mouth Is Important To Your Overall Health

With our new patients, we like to cover everything: periodontal screening, oral cancer screening, teeth and bite X-rays, and periodontal probing. We learn the whole story of the patient before developing a treatment plan. The treatment plan should be based on the patient's goals as well as the patient's current dental health. It is important to understand the patient's goals because everyone has different goals. Sometimes we need to educate our patients if their goals are unhealthy. Some 30-year-old patients come into the office and tell me, "I'm just going to pull out all of my teeth like my grandmother did." Well, that was in the 1960s.

In 2015, we can do better things for you. You do not need to go that route unless you want to. Education is so important.

Since dentists are the only ones taking care of your mouth, part of our job is to look for changes in the tissue that can indicate pre-cancerous or cancerous cells. At every visit, we perform an oral cancer screening by examining the tissues, the tongue, and the lateral borders. Oral cancer is not that common, but it can be sneaky. It can look like many different things. It can appear white or red, so we look for any type of change in the tissue, including color and texture.

Our office is proactive. We either use a brush biopsy to check suspicious tissue to make sure it is normal and healthy, or we do a traditional biopsy for anything that looks questionable. Oral screenings require ongoing exams for our patients to make sure that we do not see anything that is different or changing. This is especially true if your background or habits put you at a higher risk for oral cancer, such as patients who smoke, chew tobacco, or have a family history of cancer. If we detect or suspect oral cancer, I send that patient to the oral surgeon. As dentists, we look at your mouth at least twice a year, provided that the patient comes in for regular dental checkups. Physicians may look in the throat or mouth, but they are not looking at all of the tissues. We actually move the tongue and look at everything with a nice bright light. It is our job to make sure.

There are other things that you can see in the mouth that aren't seen in the body as quickly. Generally, HIV is detected first in the mouth, because there is a certain type of mouth lesion that people with HIV develop. We can detect diabetes in the mouth more quickly than through blood work. We may see something that other doctors didn't and tell you, "Go get your blood work done.

We're going to have to check this." That might also apply to Sjögren's syndrome or Hashimoto's, etc. Oral healthcare goes far beyond teeth and gums.

Not many physicians and primary doctors are looking at the teeth. While we receive the occasional referral, I'm not sure that other doctors are looking at the whole picture. For example, in knee replacement surgery, problems come up after the doctor fails to diagnose the patient's gum disease as an infection. A patient with gum disease can get an infection in the bloodstream that causes the new knee to fail. Only within the last two years, orthopedists have begun to refer patients to the dentist to be checked before surgeons would agree to perform knee replacements. However, we were already seeing failures due to the bacteria in the mouth; nobody ever looked in patients' mouths before they did the surgery.

There is also a strong connection between oral health, heart disease, and certain types of cancers. There are markers in the mouth. A particular DNA test in the sulcus of the tooth will tell us the markers for certain types of diseases, such as hypertension, atherosclerosis, and liver cancer. Unfortunately, these diagnostic tests are not being performed across the board in the dental field. New tests are available for investigating other conditions by checking the crevicular fluids in the mouth. However, these tests are also not widely done at this point. I am not sure why, since the crevicular fluid test is collected via an easy cotton probe, and the test also reviews several bodily problems besides tooth issues. The tests are probably dictated by insurance companies, who do not want to pay for anything new.

Gum disease is another important issue which can affect much more than the health of your mouth; around 75% of the population has some form of gum disease. Today, there are many different ways to treat gum disease, from in-office laser treatments to tooth replacement in cases of extensive gum disease. Gum disease is like diabetes; it's important to catch it early and then manage it. Since it never goes away completely, patients need to manage the gum disease to avoid experiencing bone loss around the tooth that leads to premature tooth loss. I like to begin discussing gum disease as early as possible, especially with patients in their 30s and 40s. I want them to understand why they need to be aware of gum disease and their mouth's condition, so that they do not lose their teeth prematurely.

The early stages of gum disease show in mouth inflammation. The gums bleed when you touch them. The gum tissue is unhealthy and inflamed. At that point, gum disease is very easily treatable. Generally, you're seeing the result of a lack of dental care. People are not doing very well with their homecare or haven't been to the dentist in a very long time. They may be brushing but not well. If they are flossing, they are not flossing properly. When someone shows early to moderate stages of gum disease, with a little bit of bone loss, it is important to begin treatment right away. These stages of gum disease are still easily treatable if we begin treatments right away.

With more moderate gum disease, in which the tooth loss has progressed to the point of loose or moving teeth, aggressive treatments must be performed. When a patient reports that his or her teeth are moving, this typically indicates a more severe stage of gum disease; the teeth may need to be splinted. A variety of things may need to be done to stabilize the teeth, but the prognosis is not as good with moderate or advanced gum disease.

With advanced gum disease, all of the teeth may fall out. The gum disease has attacked the bone; the bone is now missing and so the teeth are moving and falling out prematurely. In these types of cases, the teeth must be removed and replaced with an implant or denture. More severe cases mean the patient has waited a little too long to get the best results.

Catching gum disease and treating it in its early stages gives the patient the best chance for a good result. In the early stages of gum disease, treatment is likely to be more successful. With moderate to advanced stages of gum disease, there is less bone to work with, so there are fewer options for treatment. However, even in later stages of gum disease, we are still fairly successful at treating it and helping the patient to maintain a healthy mouth afterward.

Pregnancy is another example of your oral health affecting or being affected by your overall health condition. Pregnancy hormones do affect gum tissue. Typically, there will be more inflammation during pregnancy. Pregnant women need extra cleanings during pregnancy because the mouth is subject to those hormones, which make the gums more inflamed. Women have told me, "When I was pregnant, I lost a tooth." I have not found that to be true, but pregnant women do suffer from inflamed gums and more gum problems than tooth problems. Pregnancy definitely affects the hormones and the gum tissue in a negative way. You must be on top of keeping your teeth and gums clean and maintaining your regular dentist visits during pregnancy so that the mouth will stay healthy.

Sick Of Dentures: You Have More Than One Option

Patients who have been wearing dentures for many years are now looking for options. Denture issues are related to changes in your bone structure over time. Eventually, dentures start to move, they don't fit as well as your natural teeth, and they make it difficult to chew your food or speak. With dental implants, you can fit a partial denture to the implant to prevent it from moving. This is often helpful for patients who may not have the money to do an entire dental restoration with implants. Rather than having an ill-fitting denture, two or four implants can help to hold the denture in place so that it does not move. This is a good thing for patients who have been wearing dentures and have had changes in the bone since their dentures were made. The partial denture fitted to an implant will fit better and stay in place. The person will be able to speak better, chew better, and feel better about his or her appearance. Patients have many options to choose from when dealing with implants. They can have one implant all the way up to 32 implants, a bridge that sits on two implants, or a denture that sits on two implants. They can have a fixed bridge that sits on four to six implants. A patient will come into the office to discuss every possible option for his or her specific situation. Unlike a knee replacement, in which the knee comes out and a new one is put in its place, dentistry is personalized. We can replace one tooth or 20 teeth. It is all about options that are customized to each patient.

Pediatric Dentistry

I hear patients say, "They're just baby teeth" as a reason they do not worry about taking their young child to the dentist. Baby teeth are very important and do many things. They allow the child to chew, but they also hold the space for the permanent teeth. We like to see kids at an early age so that we can monitor growth and maintain healthy teeth. Keeping those primary baby teeth cavity-free so that they stay in the mouth allows the permanent teeth to erupt in the proper place.

The best thing you can do to prepare your child for the dental visit is not to prepare them. Many parents impart their fear on the child before the child arrives. Do not prepare the child for the dental visit because when you are preparing them, you tend to say things like, "You don't need to worry." What does the child do? They start to worry. "Well, she told me not to worry. I should probably worry." In our office, the first visit is a fun visit. Kids get a little ride in the chair. They get a little toy when they leave. Coming back for another visit is not a big issue. The first visit is usually just some X-rays, a cleaning, and some oral hygiene instructions.

We use air abrasion rather than using drills for cavities in children. When a mom tells her child, "The shot's not going to hurt," she unnecessarily freaks out her child because the child is not going to get a shot. Air abrasion uses small particles and air to remove a cavity and it is pain free. Let your child come into the office and let the dentist and the dental team help the child through the visit, so that the child can have a positive experience. We explain what we are doing and show them so there are no surprises. We discuss plaque, what that does to their teeth, and how that makes cavities. We watch them brush and show them proper techniques.

My Practice: Treating Multiple Generations

In our practice, we see everybody. We have four generations of patients in many families, from the little ones to Grandma. It is nice to be able to do everything for the whole family and help kids become good dental patients. Peaceful and relaxing dental visits are our goal. If we can make it a fun experience, everyone enjoys coming to the dentist. We have many kids tell us, "I can't wait to go to the dentist! When's my appointment?" It's a success to have patients who look forward to coming to the dentist. They understand why they come. They are doing a good job at home, and coming to the dentist is a positive thing for them instead of a negative, painful, and uncomfortable experience.

What we want to avoid is a patient with clenched, white knuckles. That is a clear sign of stress. We want to give children a good, positive foundation so they don't turn into adults who arrive with white knuckles because of a bad childhood experience. If we cannot train them as kids, we want to replace their bad experiences as kids or adults with good and comfortable experiences. We want them to think, "Oh, now it's more modern, more comfortable, and I can have a better experience." We have had many dental-phobic patients who needed sedation just to have an initial cleaning; after a few visits, they were able to come into the offices for a cleaning without any sedation.

It is important for me to help patients overcome their fear of dentists. Five or six years ago, they were too afraid to have X-rays, much less a cleaning, but now they come into the office for their cleaning every three months and don't need anything to make them feel comfortable. They look forward to the visit because they are not afraid. Many of our patients are dental converts who have gone from fearing the thought of a dental visit to being regular patients who are happy to come to our office. That is a wonderful feeling. Dentistry is a very rewarding profession. Every day is something different. I can help someone get out of pain, be healthier, or dramatically change their appearance.

One of the best rewards that motivates me is the smile makeover that we do. When you hand the patient the mirror and the patient begins to cry because they are overcome by what they see, you know that you have made a positive change in that person's life. Off the top of my head, I can think of half a dozen patients who were literally overwhelmed when we handed them the mirror. They said, "My goodness, I can't believe it! Now I can smile." To me, the most rewarding part of my job is when we give someone a new smile and they look in the mirror and say, "Wow! I didn't think I would ever look this good. Thank you for giving me the teeth I wanted, but I never got." We do that once or twice a week.

It is not unusual for a new patient, who has come into the office looking for a smile makeover, to see a patient in the office who has already had a smile makeover. Sometimes a patient with a hygienist will overhear the new patient and ask, "Can I show her?" It is powerful when the new patient can see an actual patient who has already benefited from our smile makeover. Our patient will say, "I did this nine years ago and I love my teeth. Whatever Dr. Jacobsen says is going to be right for you. That's what I did." We have books of before-and-after photos, but nothing is better than seeing a "live" example of how our smile makeovers can change a person's life. That live testimonial is better than anything I can say and is worth a thousand pictures.

Some of my clients love to tell their stories to potential clients when they are in the office. One patient always says, "I did this right before my son got married, and now I have all these beautiful photos." One recent patient, whose daughter recently got married, said this: "My ex-wife saw my beautiful smile. It was so nice to be able to look so good and have those pictures." Many patients are in that age bracket; their children are getting married, and they want to look good at the wedding, so they come into the office to change their smile. Others might be going to a class reunion and want to improve their smile before seeing old friends. They all say the same thing, "I should have done it 20 years ago."

I cannot tell you how rewarding it is to help people. I became a dentist in part because I had a love for science, and my dentist took the time to share the love of dentistry with me when I was young. I continue to practice dentistry because I love helping people feel better about themselves and maintain good oral health. I love my profession, I love dentistry! It is great to have a job that lets you feel so good about helping people, and you can see the results of your work when your patients smile back at you.

(This content should be used for informational purposes only. It does not create a doctor-patient relationship with any reader and should not be construed as medical advice. If you need medical advice, please contact a doctor in your community who can assess the specifics of your situation.)

2

THE IMPORTANCE OF GOOD DENTAL HEALTH TO YOUR OVERALL HEALTH & HAPPINESS

by Patricia Wu, D.M.D.

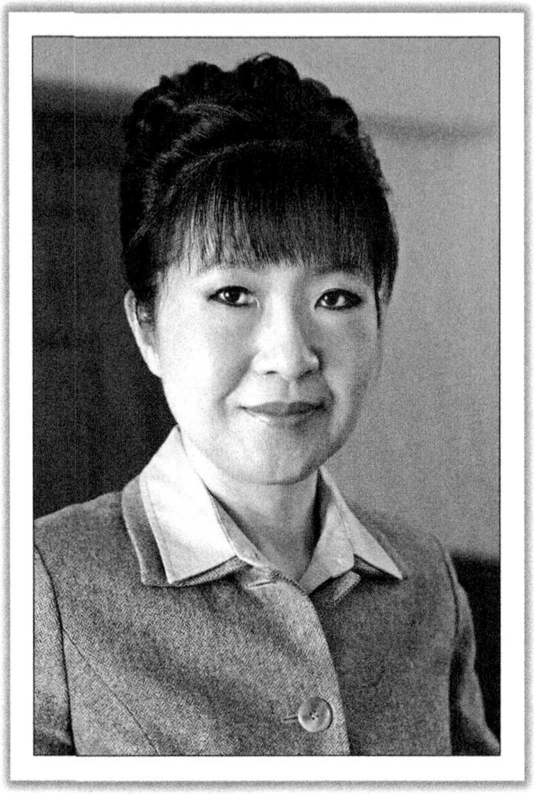

Patricia Wu, D.M.D.

Patricia Wu, D.M.D., P.C.
Malden, Massachusetts
www.mymaldendentist.com

Dr. Wu graduated with honors from Boston University Goldman School Of Dental Medicine, where she received her Doctorate in Dental Medicine (DMD) and received the prestigious award from the American College Of Prosthodontics for outstanding achievement in the study of prosthodontics.

Dr. Wu has been a general dentist since 1998. Dr. Wu is unique in her ability to connect with patients and known for giving the highest level of personal attention to her patients. Her focus on patient education has helped patient's perception about modern dentistry. She is a motivator with the gift of being able to influence others in a positive way.

Dr. Wu's vision of dentistry is very simple, to create a center of excellence for dental care with quality, integrity, ethics, and comfort. Due to her exceptional patient services and excellence in dentistry, she and her team was Patch Readers' Choice award winner for the Best Dentist in the city of Malden. She also has been recognized in the "Guide To America's Top Dentist" by Consumers' Research Council Of America for the last six years.

Dr. Wu has dedicated and committed to serve as a mentor for future dentists in Boston University Goldman School Of Dental Medicine through active participation in the APEX program for the last fourteen years. She was also once a columnist for the Malden Observer newspaper.

Dr. Wu is a member of the American Dental Association, American Academy Of Cosmetic Dentistry, Academy Of Laser Dentistry, Massachusetts Dental Society, and the East Middlesex Dental Society Of Massachusetts.

The Importance of Good Dental Health To Your Overall Health & Happiness

Coming To The United States

I was born and grew up in Taiwan. I was well loved by my parents and three sisters. As a family, we have a very close relationship and are always supportive of each other.

I'm pleased that my parents were very serious about their children getting the most out of their education, from the time that we were small girls. They did whatever they could to help us get a higher education. They constantly inspired us to reach our highest potential. They were wonderful parents, though very strict. They didn't (and still don't) allow us to take anything for granted.

I really appreciate my parents' belief in us, their constant encouragement and support, and their commitment to discipline. It was that mindset which led me to become and remain a strong woman and a competitor in my profession. The way that I was raised still helps me to always strive for the best in myself.

In September of 1987, my life changed forever. My parents, my sisters, and my brother-in-law had such faith and hope in me, they bought me a one-way plane ticket. I flew alone to the United States in order to pursue my dream. That was the first time I had ever left my family and my country.

Though I was quite young, I was not afraid. I didn't try to think too much about the fact that I was in a strange land, all by myself, with only two pieces of luggage to call my own. I began my journey in the U.S. by landing in Georgia to pursue my master's degree, and twenty-eight years have passed since then. Besides the two pieces of luggage, I also brought my guts and my brain, my dreams and my belief—and started on a journey that has brought me to where I am today.

WHY DENTISTRY?

Twenty years ago, eight years after my arrival here in the United States, I decided to change my career and enter dental school, as I would like to utilize my gift from God and rise to the challenge of pursuing an even more advanced course of education and to advance myself to the next level of my life. I had worked in the healthcare environment for several years, and I saw the dental profession as a combination of health science and art. I am passionate about health science, I am an artist, I love people, and I also love being a doctor; that was one of my childhood dreams. Since dentistry is a complex art, I thought I would fit very well in the dental profession. I was very confident that I would enjoy dentistry very much, and I proved to myself I was right.

WHAT SETS ME APART FROM OTHER DENTISTS?

My philosophy about dentistry is to be evergreen—continually striving to grow as a dentist. I work hard to provide my patients' comfort, satisfaction, and safety, while providing patients with the healthy gums and teeth that contribute toward their quality of life. Those are the top priorities in my practice. We deliver high standards of dental care with honesty, excellence, and integrity within an exceptional environment specially designed and created for both our patients and our staff.

Our commitment to learning and excellence shaped the operations of our dental office, as the team strives to invest in continual professional training. In order to provide state-of-the-art techniques, procedures, and materials, to pursue all the best that dentistry has to offer our patients, we need to stay ahead of the learning curve. We do that religiously. Our mission is to improve our patients' quality of life by helping them keep their teeth for a lifetime, while restoring and maintaining their beautiful smiles. We continue to learn and take our time with our patients in a relaxed, caring atmosphere, knowing that the work we do with our patients will last. And the patients will love what we do for them.

Our goal is to establish a long-term relationship based on trust with every patient who comes to our practice. I like to treat my patients as my family, and fortunately, many of my loyal patients treat me as family as well. Not only am I a general entist for my patients, I'm also their family dentist. So, allow your dentist to embrace you as part of his or her family. Give your dentist an opportunity to get to know you beyond just a dental level; your emotions are important and affect your health. Open up about things other than your current dental problem. You will be surprised what your dentist can do for you other than just treating your mouth.

I've always been very grateful for my strong healthcare background prior to beginning my dental career, since it provided me with a solid training in observation, communication, and people skills. Beyond mere medical knowledge, I value the experience of working in general healthcare as one of the strengths that sets me apart from other dentists. This strength enhances my ability to perform as a dentist, but it also makes me more sensitive to my patients' other potential health issues over and above their oral and dental problems.

My observation of each one of our patients begins the moment that I greet them in the waiting room. Since I believe in treating each of my patients as an entire person, when I meet with a patient, I don't just look at their mouth. Before doing a total oral exam, I take the time to review all of their medical history. I visually inspect them from head to toe. A review of medical history can help your dentist stay informed regarding your overall health, medications, medical treatments, and any illness that may impact your dental health. It's very important for patients to know that a thorough review of their personal medical history with their dentist is necessary. The more that your dentist knows about your physical condition, the better he or she will be able to help you.

Sometimes, from my visual inspection of a patient sitting in the chair, I find clues about their potential health issues. These can include skin cancer, thyroid disease, severe anemia, and even Parkinson's disease. I always share my observations with my patients, and I advise them to immediately consult with their primary physician if I notice something troubling. I appreciate that my patients take my advice seriously, and ultimately, it has helped to save their own lives. Keeping in mind that all of their personal medical and dental information is confidential, patients should have no fears about sharing information which might impact their dental health.

THE FUTURE OF DENTISTRY

Within the last century, human life expectancy has almost doubled, and the overall quality of life has improved. Some of the changes have had a positive impact on dentistry. For example, there's been an increased emphasis on oral hygiene, fluoridation, and diet improvements, not to mention easy access to health-related information via computers linked to the Internet. The over-65 population retaining their own teeth has increased along with the emphasis on keeping any of their original teeth rather than pulling them out. People now come to see dentists for reasons besides just wanting to relieve their toothache. They also now have a desire to restore the functions of their teeth to retain their teeth for a lifetime. This makes their other bodily systems work better and improves their smile so that they can look good.

Overall, the U.S. population is more educated about their oral health than ever before, especially regarding the link between oral disease and systemic disease. People now place an increased value on the positive impact of a beautiful smile on their quality of life. Because of this change, dental health will improve. Patients will want more data and information on dental health and treatment options. Dentists are seeing and will continue to see the integration of dentistry with comprehensive healthcare as we are treating patients; we're no longer just treating their teeth, their gums, or their mouth. In other words, we will see an increased focus on the link between oral health and overall health.

We will also see an increase in the implementation of technological advances. Digitalization in dental practice enables us to use a computer-assisted technology approach for better diagnosis, treatment and faster services. In the future, we will see an increase in dental clinicians using laser technology, which has revolutionized the way that doctors practice in dentistry. Going forward, more dentists will use lasers to perform more procedures, such as laser-assisted periodontal therapy. Laser assistance can improve the results of Phase One periodontal therapy.

We will also see continued improvement in materials used in dentistry to get better treatment results and to improve the longevity of a dental restoration. In many ways, we are seeing the future of dentistry every day.

The Importance Of Dental X-Rays

I focus on thorough oral exams, which include checking the overall health of a patient's teeth, gums, bite and potential TMJ issues, and performing an oral cancer screening, We also take routine checkup x-rays. Dental X-rays are a critically important step in the diagnosis of dental disease, especially in detecting oral problems that are invisible to the eye. Many oral diseases cannot be detected or even diagnosed on the sole basis of a visual or a physical examination. Sometimes tooth decay develops between the teeth or under an existing restoration. Dentists need to rely on x-rays to know the distance between tooth decay and the nerve.

X-rays can also alert your dentist to the existence of supernumerary teeth (i.e., extra teeth), along with a host of other problems: missing teeth, impacted or un-erupted teeth, tooth fractures, periodontal disease, tartar below the gum line, lesions in the jawbone, abscesses of the teeth or gums, awkward tooth positions, root configurations, root fragments, foreign bodies, and some types of tumors. X-rays can also shed light on child-related dental issues, such as the development of wisdom teeth, oral-facial growth and development. X-rays help dentists to see a better, more complete picture. A dental X-ray can also inform the dentist of changes in the patient's soft and hard tissues.

Many patients are concerned about the need for dental X-rays, mainly due to safety-related fears about radiation exposure. It's important for them to know that the dental X-ray radiation to which a patient is exposed is fairly small compared to the benefits that an X-ray provides in aiding a diagnosis or guiding a treatment plan.

Truthfully, people encounter radiation every day just by living on this planet. This is known as background radiation that occurs naturally such as cosmic rays from the sun, the stars, and terrestrial radiation from the earth itself. We are also exposed to radiation from naturally occurring radon in the air. According to the American Nuclear Society, a patient who goes through a dental X-ray is exposed to only 0.005 mSv of radiation. This is a small amount of radiation exposure, compared to (roughly) 3.2 mSv of exposure that the average American receives annually from sources that occur naturally in the environment. In fact, the average American receives more radiation from sitting in front of a television over a period of one year than from a routine dental X-ray. For your information, you are exposed to 10.00 mSv of radiation from abdomen/pelvis or whole body CT scans, according the American Nuclear Society.

People receive far more radiation from medical CT scans than from a routine dental X-ray. However, the public doesn't seem to show as much concern for CT scans. Patients who will refuse to take a dental X-ray with low radiation will not refuse to take a CT scan with a lot higher amount of radiation based on their medical doctor's order. Patients don't mind receiving constant excess radiation from intense sunlight to tan their skin at the beach, but they worry over a dental X-ray. We really don't know where the bias is coming from, but it isn't a logical one.

The bottom line is that dentists need a proper diagnostic tool to make an accurate, definitive diagnosis, just as medical doctors need diagnostic tools. I would not be able to treat a patient in my office for the first time if they refused to take an X-ray unless they brought in a recent copy of a usable X-ray from their previous dentist. Baseline images are very important to patients and their dentists. Without X-ray images as references for dental procedures, your dentist is blindfolded in treating you. That's not safe for you. So, you really don't want to put your dentist in that situation.

In my office, we work to help eliminate the concerns surrounding dental X-rays by using equipment and techniques that are designed to limit the body's exposure to radiation. Every precaution is taken by dental professionals to ensure that a patient's radiation exposure is as low as reasonably achievable. For example, the use of four protective tools (lead apron, lead thyroid collar, E- or F-speed film, or digital X-rays) all help to limit exposure. In my office, we use digital X-rays. Digital radiograph devices allow our patients to receive 80 to 90 percent less radiation than is needed to expose conventional film and its images. Digital images are instantly available from the radiograph. Instead of making duplicates, we can email your radiographs anywhere that they need to go or simply print them out. We usually don't take X-rays on a pregnant patient unless there is a specific dental emergency.

There are no state laws governing the frequency of X-rays, but there are standards of care that dentists utilize based on clinical evaluation, risk factors, and established recommendations to determine X-ray frequency. These recommendations are subject to the dentist's clinical judgment and may not apply to every patient. Each dental office may have a different routine dental X-ray schedule. If you have any concerns about your child's health or your own oral health in regards to a dental X-ray, then don't hesitate to speak with your dentist. However, it's a good idea to trust your dentist's clinical judgment in providing you with the best diagnosis and treatment while maintaining your safety in regard to the dental X-ray.

New Weapon Of Bacterial Destruction: Laser Assisted Periodontal Therapy

According to recent findings from the Centers for Disease Control and Prevention (CDC), one out of every two American adults, aged 30 and over, has some type of periodontal disease. In adults 65 and older, the prevalence rate increases to 70 percent. Periodontal diseases are infections that affect the tissue and the bone that supports your teeth. In the early stage, this disease is chronic and silent, so you don't even feel it. (That's why regular dental check-ups and periodontal examinations are so very important.) Periodontal disease is an ongoing inflammation caused by bacteria that live in plaque. Plaque is the sticky, colorless film that is always forming on your teeth. Plaque contains bacteria that can irritate and inflame your gums and make them red, tender, and likely to bleed. This condition is called gingivitis.

Gingivitis can be reversed if the plaque is removed. You can do this simply by improving your oral care at home, brushing and flossing twice a day, and having your teeth cleaned regularly at the dental office. If you don't get rid of gingivitis, it can turn into periodontitis, which involves progressive loss of the bone that supports the teeth. This condition is irreversible; if left untreated, it can lead to the loosening and subsequent loss of your teeth.

Tooth loss is not the only potential problem posed by periodontal disease. Studies have suggested that there is a link between periodontal diseases and other health concerns, such as heart disease, diabetes, stroke, and increased risk during pregnancy. Early detection and treatment are the keys to successfully controlling disease.

Periodontal treatments depend upon the type and severity of the disease. If the disease is caught at a very early stage and no damage has been done, you may simply be given instructions on improving your daily oral hygiene. Even with these measures, some patients develop more severe periodontal disease that must be treated.

Conventional initial therapy is called "scaling and root planing." This is sometimes referred to as "periodontal cleaning" or "deep cleaning." It removes plaque and tartar build-up beneath the gum line. This procedure allows the gum tissue to heal. In more severe cases, if the dental pockets don't heal after initial therapy, periodontal surgery may be needed.

Many people think that gum therapy is a painful procedure with a long recovery time. Those perceptions tend to make patients shy away from seeking help from a dentist to treat their periodontal problem before it becomes worse. Fortunately, laser gum therapy is starting to change that perception. The soft tissue lasers have become our new weapon of bacterial destruction to help our patients battle against periodontal disease. The laser energy removes the diseased tissue on the inside of the pocket, significantly reduces bacteria, and provides an optimal environment for speeding the healing process.

The soft tissue laser, when used in conjunction with a conventional scaling and root planing treatment, is documented to be far more effective over the long term than the scaling and root planing procedure alone. In other words, it improves periodontal therapy and greatly reduces the need for a surgery to treat gum disease. Other benefits include a reduced need for local anesthesia, the immediate cessation of gum bleeding, few to no post-operative discomforts, and a faster recovery time.

We have added soft tissue diode laser to our practice in order to offer assisted periodontal therapy to our patients. This technology offers a wonderful way to encourage acceptance of periodontal therapy, both in new patients and current patients who have been avoiding treatment due to fear of pain.

WHAT CAN YOU DO ABOUT TOOTH SENSITIVITY?

Tooth sensitivity is a common name for "dentin hypersensitivity." Tooth sensitivity is best described as a short, sharp pain. Some people describe the feeling as twinges or "zings" initiated by hot or cold food and drinks, sweet or acidic foods, breathing in cool air, or even by something or someone touching the teeth. Tooth sensitivity is one of the most common complaints among dental patients. Some patients even require an emergency visit to address the pain. Tooth sensitivity is not a disease but rather an oral condition that affects approximately half the population.

Understanding our tooth structure will help us to understand tooth sensitivity. In healthy teeth, enamel protects the underlying layer of dentin; the gums protect the roots of the teeth. The roots also have another covering, an outer layer called "cementum." When the enamel is worn down or damaged, or when gums have receded, the cementum is lost, and then the dentin becomes exposed. The dentin layer contains thousands of tiny tubules (dentin tubules) that are only visible when examined under a microscope. They run through the dentin layer and connect to the nerves in the center of the tooth, called the "pulp." These dentinal tubules contain plasma-like biological fluid.

When dentinal tubules are exposed after enamel or cementum loss, due to a variety of factors, the flow or movement of the biological fluid is increased by either cold or hot air blasts, sugary or sour stuff, or forces such as touching the tooth with a dental instrument. These things acting upon the tooth irritate the nerves inside the tooth, triggering the pain we understand as tooth sensitivity.

The most important factor of dentin hypersensitivity is exposed dentin that happens as a result of gum recession with the exposure of root surfaces and loss of a cementum layer. It also can be as a result of loss of enamel associated with tooth wear. Gum recession can be a sign of long-term trauma caused by excessive or forceful tooth brushing, improper tooth-brushing technique, or brushing with an abrasive toothpaste and/or hard bristled tooth brush. It also can be a sign of chronic gum disease.

The causes of tooth wear can be related to chewing tobacco, teeth grinding or clenching, or erosion related to excessive acid (e.g., over-consumption of acidic foods and drinks, acid reflux disease, or bulimia). Other identifiable factors contributing to tooth sensitivity include dental decay, chipped or cracked teeth, fractured restorations, restorations with a margin leakage, or tooth whitening. Some people get temporary tooth sensitivity from whitening or other dental procedures, such as fillings. If you have tooth sensitivity associated with these factors, you should see your dentist for an evaluation as soon as possible. This can be a serious problem, and a dental procedure may be required to address the sensitivity.

Dentin hypersensitivity can be a complex issue. It's best diagnosed by a thorough dental screening, a clinical and radiographic exam, and a review of the patient's dental history. The strategies for managing the tooth sensitivity condition can be quite varied. There's no gold standard treatment that works for everybody. Allow your dentist to determine the most likely cause of your tooth sensitivity and the best solution for your particular situation.

Once your dentist determines that the cause of tooth sensitivity does not require a restorative dental procedure (fillings, crowns, root canal treatment, or gum treatment), treatment options can be a relatively simple matter. Either they can be applied in-office by your dentist or dental hygienist or carried out at home after you get an over-the-counter medication or prescription. For high-level tooth sensitivity, your dentist may recommend in-office treatments that include a fluoride treatment. Either fluoride gel with tray applications or fluoride varnish can be directly painted on the exposed dentin or root surface to strengthen the area and block the exposure of the dentinal tubules. Your dentist may also apply a desensitizing agent to block the dentinal tubules, which blocks off the transmission of sensation from the tooth to the nerve.

For low-level tooth sensitivity, at-home treatments can be effective: eating a healthy diet, avoiding or limiting the consumption of acidic foods and drinks, and good oral hygiene practices (flossing, brushing twice a day). For sensitive teeth, it's an especially good idea to use a non-traumatic tooth-brushing technique with a soft-bristled toothbrush and non-abrasive desensitizing toothpaste. Your dentist may also prescribe a brush-on fluoride gel or dental paste with a higher fluoride level. You can spread a thin layer of this gel or dental paste onto the exposed dentin or root surface at bedtime to provide you with extra protection. This product should be used on a regular basis to be able to see the therapeutic effect. If you have underlying medical conditions such as acid reflux or bulimia, you should seek medical treatment to stop the erosion of your teeth and eventually address your tooth sensitivity from these medical conditions. If your tooth sensitivity is caused by tooth wear from grinding and/or clenching, you should have your dentist make a night guard appliance to wear when you sleep at night. Prevention is the key. Prevention is the most cost-effective treatment option for tooth sensitivity.

Some patients may wonder if sensitivity after a filling is normal. Some sensitivity is normal after a tooth has been worked on, especially after any kind of filling, from small to large—and especially if there has been tooth decay. As bacteria enters the pulp from tooth decay, the tooth becomes sensitive because the tissue is irritated and any work done on the tooth can irritate it further. The tooth should improve, usually within days; some patients may take longer for recovery, even up to several months. The decay could have been very deep, close to the pulp of the tooth. As long as the tooth sensitivity gradually improves, there should be no cause for worry.

If the sensitivity persists after a deep filling, it's an indicator that the tooth is not recovering from this situation and may possibly need a root canal procedure. If the tooth is sensitive to biting after a filling is done, it may only mean that you need a simple bite adjustment. So, when you experience sensitivity after a dental procedure, call your dentist for an evaluation to see if any further procedure needs to be done.

Creating Your Own Happiness With A Beautiful Smile

A smile makeover does not necessarily involve the entire mouth, nor does it always mean a great expense. We do smile makeovers for our patients every day in our office. Smile makeovers can be small procedures, like a tooth-colored filling, or they can be very involved procedures, such as whole mouth reconstruction.

There are several popular treatment options for a smile makeover: tooth-colored fillings, tooth whitening, tooth movement (braces or Invisalign®), crown lengthening for a gummy smile, enamel shaping, and/or veneers. Sometimes, a bridge or a dental implant will also be considered. Treatment may be more affordable than you think.

Tooth whitening is one of the most in-demand, popular cosmetic procedures requested in my office. It is my passion to help my patients get the whiter teeth they have always dreamed about. Age doesn't matter as long as you are a good candidate for the process of whitening. Not only do white teeth look good and enhance your smile, they make you feel more confident about your appearance. I have seen this result in my office many times. The oldest patient who has asked for teeth whitening in my office was an elderly female patient who was 84 years old. She had been dreaming about a whiter smile for her entire life. She has been whitening her teeth for four years, and she is very happy with her smile. That matters to the patient, and it matters to us.

Not everyone will get the same whitening results, and not everyone has the same personal expectations. We are very careful in the selection and the strength of the whitening agents. We must also consider the length of exposure of our patient's teeth to whitening agents, the selection of whitening techniques, the patient's compliance level, and the intrinsic versus extrinsic stain of their existing teeth. These factors will show in the ultimate success of the process. It's important to understand the patient's expectations from the process in the end. We require patients to have a thorough oral exam prior to a whitening procedure, as we want to make sure their gums and teeth are in reasonable condition.

Two common potential side effects are thermal hypersensitivity and gingival irritation. It's good to know that there is no cumulative or permanent side effect, because both of these effects are reversible.

The whitening frequency will vary based on your needs and color preferences. Whitening durations vary from person to person. Certain factors (food, drinks, tobacco use, age, medication) can affect the longevity of your results. There are several types of whitening therapies that may be done in-office or at home. My patients like in-office whitening more than take-home treatments because they have faster results and we do all of the work for them. We use a couple popular whitening systems: Zoom!® In-Office Whitening System and Sinsational Smile® In-Office Whitening System. Sinsational Smile® uses an LED accelerating light that helps to activate the ingredients of the whitening gel at a faster rate. This results in a bright smile and whiter teeth in less time—only 20 minutes.

The best time to have your teeth whitened is right after your teeth have been professionally cleaned. We frequently schedule our patients for Sinsational Smile® on their hygiene visits. Patients stay for another 20 minutes after their cleaning to get their teeth whitened. None of our patients have experienced tooth sensitivity from these whitening procedures, but this procedure gives you a more subtle shade change than others.

Zoom!® In-Office Whitening is a procedure designed to lighten the color of your teeth using a combination of hydrogen peroxide gel and a specially-designed ultraviolet lamp. It requires more chair time, with three 15-minute sessions, but it's a very powerful whitening system. It may be a better option for a patient whose teeth have dark grey shades or thicker enamel and are more difficult to whiten. Some patients do experience temporary tooth sensitivity with these treatments, but for most patients, that sensitivity goes away within 24 to 72 hours. We see good whitening results with both whitening systems. Your dentist will help you to decide which system is more suitable for your teeth.

To help more patients find their brightest smile and make their dream come true in a very affordable way, we established the Whitening for Life Club in my office. Patients who have had a whitening procedure done in our office get an invitation to join this club. They get a free whitening gel twice a year as long as they maintain their six-month hygiene visit to make sure their gums and teeth are in good shape for continual whitening.

When patients ask if they should whiten their teeth, I always tell them—as long as it makes them happy or will change their life in a positive way—to go ahead and do it. Be sure that your periodontal condition and your teeth are in good standing before you whiten your teeth.

Why Old Dental Fillings Need To Be Replaced

Dental fillings, also called dental restorations, may last many years before they need to be replaced. However, there are a number of reasons your fillings may need to be replaced. Constant stress from chewing, grinding, and crunching teeth may eventually cause a filling to wear down, chip, or fracture. A filling may also need to be replaced if the surrounding tooth structure becomes decayed. A worn-out filling will leave a gap at the filling, providing an entry point for decay-causing bacteria. If the seal between the tooth and the filling breaks down, bacteria and foreign particles can work their way in between the worn-out filling and the tooth and cannot be easily removed with a toothbrush or by other methods.

Decay may also develop along the edge of the filling or underneath it. If the decay is left untreated, it can infect the nerve tissue. This often results in the need for a root canal procedure. If left untreated, decay can even lead to a fracturing of the tooth structure; some patients may lose their teeth when severe tooth fracturing occurs beyond repair. Worn fillings should be replaced before any decay begins. Don't wait until the tooth hurts, or a crack appears in the filling or in the tooth itself. A crack or an infection may make the treatment more complicated and expensive. Extensive tooth decay along an existing restoration may leave behind very little tooth structure after the decay is removed. In that case, a crown may be recommended to completely cover and protect the remaining tooth structure.

Regular dental examinations are important because problems with existing fillings can often be detected in the early stage of decay. Although you may not be able to tell that your restoration is worn out, your dentist can identify weaknesses in your dental restoration during the regular check-up. During the exam, your dentist will determine if the existing fillings are intact or if any have cracked or become worn out. Dental X-rays may be taken to find the decay under a filling or between the teeth, neither of which can be identified by simply looking at the tooth.

Choosing The Right Dentist For You And Your Family

Most people want to find a dentist they can trust, who will care for them and their family, and who has their best interests in mind. Other than the necessary credentials, it's important to look for these things:

- Look for a dentist with adequate training, experience, and special education, especially in the area of specialized services. If you have severe dental anxiety, for example, a dentist trained in sedation dentistry will be an advantage for you.

- Take advantage of any free consultation to visit the prospective dentist and their team to get a feel for the office atmosphere. Are they friendly, and courteous?
- Get advice from many sources, while understanding that nothing is guaranteed. A friend may recommend their dentist and you may find them to be a good choice, or you may not. Online reviews sometimes can be a useful source, but should not be a sole factor to decide who will be your dentist.
- Personality plays a very important role in the choice. How does the doctor's personality match yours? I think it is a very important factor. Observe the chair-side manner of the doctor and the hygienist. Does your dentist or hygienist give you enough personal attention? Going to the dentist is stressful enough. You want someone who is warm and friendly. Find an office you can connect with, where you can feel at home.
- Accessibility can also be a factor to some people. Do you prefer a dentist's location near your workplace or your home? Convenience, dental insurance, and fees—all of these can be taken into consideration.

Your Quality Of Life Counts

I have a story that addresses the quality of life related to dental care I would like to share. It is about my father. He was a very kind, caring gentleman, always with a positive attitude. We loved him deeply and so did his friends. He passed away because of uncontrolled diabetes, leading to multi-organ failure. Without forcing anything, sometimes I share my father's story with my patients to help them make a decision regarding their treatment options to improve their quality of life. My father had chronic illness for many, many years. The illness eventually affected his mouth and his teeth. By the end stage of his illness, he had lost most of his teeth.

As his illness became more severe, he was not able to easily travel anymore and had to use a wheelchair. His dentures became ill-fitting and were bothering him to the point that he could not eat well with them. He could have fixed his dentures when he was in better physical condition, but he didn't. Fortunately, there was a short period of time when his condition improved, so he was able to get to a dental clinic in Taiwan. The process of making a new set of dentures went very well. He was very happy and was looking forward to eating better with his new dentures, but unfortunately, his condition suddenly and very quickly deteriorated. My father passed away just a day before his final denture appointment. He never had a chance to wear his new dentures. We buried his dentures with him.

At that time, I was still a dental student in the U.S. I wished that I was already a dentist so that I could have offered him a new set of dentures to improve his quality of life before he passed away. Some of my patients have some sort of similar situation. I share my father's story with them so that they can really think about what is important for the life they have left. I try to emphasize the quality of their life. Why shouldn't they be enabled to enjoy their final months and years?

I told my father's story to the daughter of one of my patients (both of whom are patients of mine). Her father was 87 years old at the time and he hated to wear dentures. He had a partial denture, which he had never liked. We discussed dental implant options. Even though he was elderly, he was still a good candidate for dental implants. His daughter helped him to make the decision to go ahead with the dental implants, and the placement procedure was very successful. Afterward, he never needed to wear dentures again. He was very, very happy. He lived for another few years and I was thrilled that, as a result of the implants, he was able to enjoy a better quality of life in his final years.

Finally, this chapter is written in memory of my father for serving as a role model to me as a business owner, where his spirit has guided me through my journey. I also would like to thank my mother, my sisters, my brother-in-law, my husband, and the wonderful people whom I have met along the way who have made my dream possible. Not every person gets an opportunity to relocate to the other side of the planet to seize an opportunity to learn and pursue their dreams. It was because of that opportunity that I was able to become a dentist, a wonderful profession that allows me to pass the gift I have from God along to other people by improving the quality of life they enjoy, and helping them to increase their confidence and create their happiness in life. I am very grateful!

(This content should be used for informational purposes only. It does not create a doctor-patient relationship with any reader and should not be construed as medical advice. If you need medical advice, please contact a doctor in your community who can assess the specifics of your situation.)

3

THE IMPORTANCE OF PEDIATRIC DENTISTRY: PROVIDING A GOOD FOUNDATION FOR LIFETIME DENTAL HEALTH

by Peter Fuentes, D.M.D.

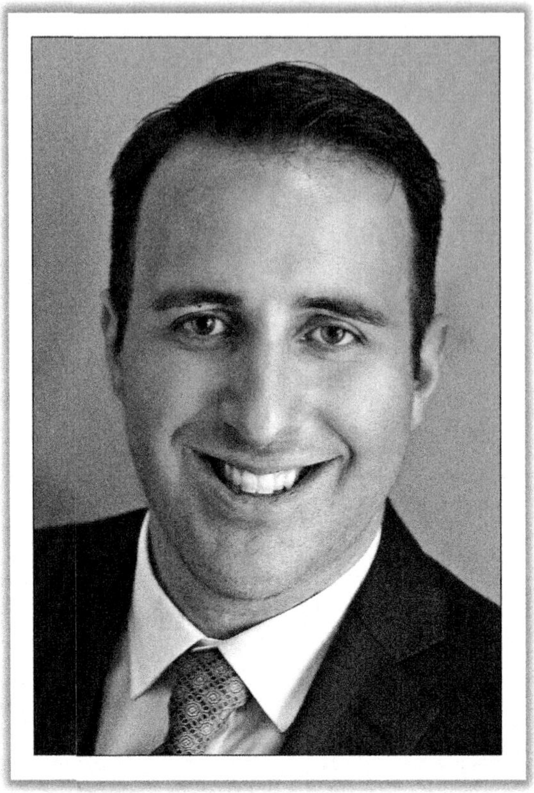

Peter Fuentes, D.M.D.

Bayonne Family Dental
Bayonne, New Jersey
www.bayonnefamilydental.com

In 2007, Dr. Peter Fuentes and his business partner and fellow dentist Salvatore Pavone, founded Dental Groups of New Jersey, which now includes multiple dental practices, several in poverty-challenged, underserved cities like Bayonne, Paterson, and East Orange. Fuentes vision for dentistry is one of outreach. Pavone and Fuentes have opened up their offices to the community, mental health facilities, nursing homes, special care facilities, as well as public and private schools. "We view our offices as a fixture in the communities. We want everyone to feel welcomed. We have buses from Senior centers bringing patients here weekly. It becomes a bit of a social hour for the residents. They bring photos, keepsakes, and often food to share with the staff." Fuentes' offices have also been vital in public health reform. They have initiated mandatory dental checkups for many of the daycares, nursery schools, as well as high schools. "We just need to make sure that these kids are being seen regularly by a dentist. Almost all dental emergencies are things that could have been prevented with routine care."

Fuentes says he was drawn to dentistry through a passion for public health. "I've always been interested in helping people in a bigger sense, more than just a one-on-one relationship with people," he says. "Dentistry is advocacy. Our job is to basically look after these kids, and oral health is just our way in the door."

Dr. Peter Fuentes graduated from Johns Hopkins University where he studied Neuroscience, and then went on to graduate from UMDNJ-New Jersey Dental. He continues to work on his Alumni Admissions board at Johns Hopkins. Currently, he holds the post as Liberty Dental's Medicaid Dental Director for the state of New Jersey. He was named "Top Dentist" By New Jersey Monthly Magazine 2012 and the recipient of Academy of Osseointegration Implant Dentist Award. He has been honored by multiple organizations for his work servicing the underprivileged population in the community.

His wife, Dr Meghan Hernandez, shares his vision and passion for dentistry. Together, they have 2 children, Isabella Rose and Erik Arturo.

THE IMPORTANCE OF PEDIATRIC DENTISTRY: PROVIDING A GOOD FOUNDATION FOR LIFETIME DENTAL HEALTH

EDUCATION WAS IMPORTANT FROM EARLY CHILDHOOD

I grew up in a small suburb in central New Jersey called Bound Brook. Mine was something of a non-traditional family. I was the son of a politically exiled father who met my mother in the United States even though their backgrounds were significantly different. My father came to this country in 1961 from Cuba, seeking political asylum following the Bay of Pigs invasion. My mother was born in this country, but spent much of her childhood in a remote, mountainous region of Italy with her family.

I went to a very small public high school—I'm being somewhat charitable when I say it was not exactly comparable to what most of my colleagues experienced. It continuously ranks in the lower third of all the public schools in the entire state of New Jersey. My high school was made up of a large population of non-English speaking Costa Rican immigrants. While very hard working, many of these students did not enter high school with the vision of attending college but rather a career in the trade industry.

My decision in favor of higher education came, for the most part, from my mother and father. The value of education was one of the lessons they drilled into me over and over again. Education was the one thing that my father was most proud of owning. He earned his Ph.D. while he was still in Havana, Cuba. When the unrest started, he came to America. He would always tell us that his education was the only thing that a government couldn't take from him. They took his family's land, they split up his family, and he left Cuba an exile. This is a very important distinction. Most stories of American immigration start with leaving poverty for the dream of employment, security, and possessions. The story of the Cuban exile is often one of leaving employment and possessions for uncertainty and poverty.

However, his education was the one thing that traveled with him which survived exile. Therefore, not surprisingly, our family mantra has become, "The most important thing you own is your education."

My brothers and I were active in many clubs and activities. I grew up playing every organized sport I could find. I played baseball, football, basketball, wrestling, tennis, and soccer. However, regardless of any achievements in athletics—no matter how big or small—in my household, those achievements were secondary to academic achievement. My parents kept us focused on our education at all times. Being the youngest of three boys, I always felt the pressure of keeping up with my successful older brothers. They became my role models for success.

The two fondest memories of my youth were being able to inform my parents of my acceptance into college and my acceptance into dental school. The pride that my parents had in me was amazing and inspiring. I honestly think if I had won an Olympic medal my parents wouldn't have been as proud. Their son was going to be a doctor. I was going to make them proud.

Furthering My Education & Choosing A Career

I attended Johns Hopkins University in Baltimore, Maryland, to study neuroscience. When I arrived, it was very humbling.

Compared to a lot of incoming freshmen, I was under-prepared. Many of my friends and old classmates arrived with 15 or 18 Advanced Placement (A.P.) credits already under their belts. We didn't have an A.P. course in my high school, so I'd never taken any A.P. tests and didn't know what one was. Going from the small pond of a public high school to a large private university institution where everybody had already distinguished themselves at the top of the academic food chain made me feel a little insignificant. It was really challenging at first. I can't tell you how much it meant to have my mother and father there behind me, pushing me along, reinforcing the benefits of hard work. I just put my head down and managed to get through every day. I was never the smartest student in school. But I was willing to outwork everyone to keep up. I spent more time in the university library the first year than I spent in my dorm room.

Around my third year at Johns Hopkins, I realized that medicine and dentistry were things that I had to pursue—I wanted to. It was a calling for me. There wasn't a moment in time, a lightbulb moment or an epiphany, when I said, "Hey, I want to be a dentist." I don't have any traumatic dental stories from my childhood. I often fantasize how great a story it would be if a dentist had saved my life as a child, or if a dentist had inspired me to go to school—but no, that didn't happen. Dentistry was an option when I was applying to school. It seemed like the profession would be a good life fit for me. I did some research and was interested. I applied and I got in. I will tell you now, with 100 percent honesty, I cannot imagine a better position for me out there in the world. I'm in love with dentistry.
Speaking of great loves, I am married to one of mine. My wife, Dr. Megan Hernandez, is also a dentist. We were never in dental school at the same time, however we attended the same university. That is my coy way of saying that I am four years her elder. We actually met later, after we'd both graduated. The first

question people ask when meeting us for the first time is, "Do you guys work together?" The answer "NO" usually arrives before the question is finished being asked. We do work together in another aspect of life: the raising of our two children. Isabella Rose and Erik Arturo are the other two loves of my life.

When we think of life-altering events, most parents would list the birth of their first child. My daughter, Isabella, was born on Christmas Eve, and it was a day I'll never forget. She came a few weeks early and we weren't quite ready. My wife and I, both doctors, were woefully unprepared for what was ahead of us. Her water broke in the middle of the night and we looked at each other and said, "What do we do?" Were we supposed to call a doctor? Spending our entire careers looking in people's mouths does not adequately prepare one for the procedures of childbirth. Since my only child birthing experiences up to that point had been played out on television, I expected this process to play out in a heartbeat. I've since joked with my friends that every television show that I've ever watched lied to me because, in Hollywood, when the mother's water breaks, the baby is delivered within minutes—in a cab, in a police car, or in a fire house. So, there I was, running around the house frantically trying to get everything together. My wife was looking at me as if I'd gone completely crazy. I'm thinking, "Oh, my gosh! I'm going to have to deliver my baby in my car." Meanwhile, my wife steps into the shower and starts shampooing her hair. In real life, babies usually work on a more reasonable timeline. My daughter arrived 14 hours after my wife rinsed out her conditioner.

My daughter is my best friend. She makes every day a little bit better. Isabella has taught me so much about patience and growth, along with some of the nuances of life—the first steps, the first word, the first time she used the fork by herself. These are just little things that, if you're not a parent, you probably won't understand (I never did). Once you are a parent, you completely understand when someone else gets excited about what non-parents see as trivial. When my daughter said "daddy" for the first time, or the first time our dog licked her and she fell into fits of giggling—those are the unexplainable joys of parenting.

BUILDING A SUCCESSFUL DENTAL PRACTICE

I graduated dental school in 2005. In 2007, with my business partner, Dr. Salvatore Pavone, we opened up our first practice in an urban setting, Union City, New Jersey; it has one of the highest population densities in the country. We were dealing with such a large population of children in the beginning that we realized these were the issues and the people who were most important to us. After that, we opened up our second location.

Fast-forward five years, and we now have had five offices open in five different major cities, some in very metropolitan areas in New Jersey. We are one of the largest dental providers in the state of New Jersey. Our offices routinely see between 80 and 100 patients a day. The majority of our patients are children and teenagers. That's where we can have the most influence in the market. We really stress diet and preventive care from the very early years up to the teen years. We have more than a dozen associate dentists who work for us providing about every dental procedure imaginable. We have root canal specialists, orthodontists, pediatric dentists, and an oral surgeon who all work for us.

We opened our office to be a community center of dentistry. Our youngest patients come into our office at 6 months of age, and we treat many patients who are in their nineties. We have redefined the art of true "family dentistry."

In these high-volume cities, we were seeing many children who were either emigrating or were first-generation immigrants from other countries in Central America, South America, the Caribbean, and the Middle East. We came to realize that the standard of care in dentistry varies greatly throughout the world. Many of our Middle Eastern patients are six and seven years old, but they have never seen a dentist before. They're drinking chocolate milk every night before bed. With many of our patients from Latin America, their parents put sugar in their milk at bedtime because they think it makes them sleep better. It's no surprise that we see increasing tooth decay in this population.

So for us—for my partner Dr. Salvatore and me—it's important to make a difference very early in life. You can't wait six or seven years to get involved and change the diet of a child. It needs to start so much earlier for many reasons. For instance, if a tooth gets pulled out too early, the child may have speech issues. Most likely, he or she will have to see an orthodontic specialist later in life. Crooked teeth arise. For us, a big portion of what we do is not only preventive dentistry—I think that's really important—but also educational dentistry. We are de facto nutritionists for a lot of these families. We are de facto pediatricians for a lot of these families. For us, dentistry is a lot more about getting to the root of the problem, understanding the psychology of patients, and honestly knowing a little about their background and where they're from. To people who were born in this country, all of this may seem like common sense, advice you've heard your whole life. In other countries and other cultures around the world, oral health is viewed much differently.

I'm very proud to have the opportunity to currently serve as one of the insurance dental directors for Medicaid in the state of New Jersey. I became the dental director mostly to have an arena in which to argue my convictions on public health and children's preventive dentistry. New Jersey has a very large population of children who are covered under Medicaid as their primary dental insurer. Part of what I've done is come up with some of the guidelines for the insurance companies in an effort to get kids into dental offices earlier and start that preventive process. This involves helping the parents to understand that their kids have dental benefits available.

I'm very proud of being a Medicaid dental director because it lets me actually have a larger-scale effect on children in New Jersey than if my influence was just one-on-one in an office. It allows me to enact policy, which encourages children and parents to be more involved with their dentists in regards to health. The rest of this chapter is a peek inside some of this policy, as well as a guideline that has been formed out of 10 years in private practice.

When To Bring Your Child To The Dentist

It still boggles my mind when parents are surprised to learn that giving their kid apple juice every single day is TERRIBLE for their teeth. The two most harmful things that cause tooth decay is sugar and acid. All juices, especially apple juice, are guilty offenders of those.

So the job of dentists is to get to parents and caretakers early. We need to help them connect the dots and realize that doing this one thing could result in widespread tooth decay. When tooth decay is so severe, sometimes it cannot be repaired and teeth need to be pulled out. This can start happening as soon as teeth are coming into a baby's mouth. That's why we make it such a priority to get kids in at 12–18 months old for check-ups—because we want to start before those problems arise. That's what separates us from a lot of other dentists. The previous mindset of many dentists was "Wait until they're three to five years old to come in." Our paradigm has shifted away from that model toward getting the initial visits done earlier. A dentist doesn't need to wait until all your baby's teeth have grown or until the child can sit in the chair calmly by himself. The choice between healthy teeth or decay can't wait that long.

Decay doesn't wait for anybody. As soon as there are teeth in the mouth, there's a risk of decay, so 12–18 months is a good time to start. If parents want to bring in their kids at 9 months, we're happy to see them as well. For us, the big change that we're trying to establish is starting routine dentistry earlier. In our 10 years of private practice, we have noticed that it actually makes a difference, which is fun. We're seeing eight- and nine-year-olds that we saw at ages one and two. These kids are cavity-free and their teeth are beautiful—yet their older siblings (who we didn't see that young) have root canals and missing teeth. The biggest difference in these siblings are earlier preventative dentistry and an earlier intervention to a healthy diet.

Friday Drinks: The Damage Of Sweets

Here's how things have changed. When I was in elementary school as a kid, we always used to get excited for Fridays in the cafeteria, because Friday was chocolate milk day—and pizza day. It was the big, exciting thing. There was always boring white milk every day. We would see the cart of milk come in on Friday and we'd all get excited. As a kid, this made Fridays the greatest day ever. Somewhere along the line, though, this has changed to many schools offering chocolate milk every day. This may not seem like such a big deal at first glance. However, it starts a pattern that is distressing to us dentists.

Now as dentists, we fight an overarching issue: we don't want to necessarily deprive our children of any sweets or anything above water and white milk. However, there is a difference between depriving children and overwhelming them with sugar. This is one of the topics we harp on. We tell our patients and their parents that there's a whole category of drinks that we call our once-a-week drinks or Friday drinks: chocolate milk, strawberry milk, fruit juices, iced tea, soda, lemonade, fruit punch, and sports drinks. Then there are two and only two everyday drinks: white milk and water. Your kids should be having those drinks every single day. Obviously, there are dietary substitutes for white milk, like soy milk or almond milk, but in general, only white milk and water should be allowed every day. Many times, parents are shocked to hear that apple juice or orange juice is not a healthy liquid alternative for children. What we inform parents is that apples and oranges are great. Apple juice and orange juice are not.

The liquid diet of young children is probably the biggest fight we have as dentists and the greatest indicator of tooth decay. Most parents have a very good handle on solid foods—what's healthy and not healthy. We never have a parent who comes into the office and says, "I give my kid a chocolate bar every single day," or "I give my kids cupcakes every day." Of course, parents know the answer to that situation is NO! Maybe they'll do cupcakes once or twice a week or let their kids have a piece of birthday cake at a birthday party here or there. Parents are fine with that idea, but the liquids are the problem at this age, because most children drink a lot more than they eat, and you can easily lose track of the drinks.

For example, a child may have a glass of orange juice for breakfast. That is sugary drink number one. Then comes lunchtime. Kids are now drinking a sweetened iced tea at lunchtime, or maybe Mom packed them a juice box if they bring their lunch. That's sugar drink number two. Then they have some chocolate milk in the afternoon. Kids are drinking three to four sugary drinks every day. The parents lose track. They say, "My kids don't drink soda." (That's always the first response we hear from parents.) That's wonderful. I'm glad to hear that, but soda's not the only drink we should worry about. The sugar content in the apple juice and juice boxes and sports drinks is astounding. When these are drunk all day long by kids, they quickly become the major culprit of tooth decay in younger children.

Educating The Parents

Now, some families may have traditions they don't break, habits from the old world which have been passed down from generation to generation or misconceptions about nutrition and health. A lot of what we do centers on education, which starts with the parents. That's where we try to get our foot in the door in this community. If we can get through to the parents and strongly impress our mindset of nutritional importance upon the parents, then the understanding becomes generational—they pass along the knowledge to their children. We can only hope it carries through to the grandchildren.

We hope that the focus becomes the standard for the many cities where we are—that we place an emphasis on early nutritional health with kids. Good nutrition is not a topic that often gets covered by pediatricians in infants and toddlers. Much of the kids' understanding comes from grandparents who are from another country, and the nutritional model that they've been following may lead to early tooth loss and decay. The grandparents may even think that tooth loss is normal—that was their reality. Now, here, they have good nutrition available all the time. For us, those are always our main issues: starting young and starting with diet. Settling those issues pays such great dividends later in life, through adolescence and the teenage years.

In our practice, we take the position that there is a larger public health issue at stake. That's the essence of the fight in our office with our patients and their families—the problem and its solution involves the entire family. Good nutrition and good diet are not the responsibilities of a three-year old. All of that falls on the parents and caretakers. The parents also fall back upon the grandparents, aunts, and uncles—whoever the caretakers may be—for reasons and explanations. "Grandma gives him this and that. Grandpa always gives him a lollipop." That's fine, but if Grandpa were allowing your son to play in traffic, you'd find a way to stop that. If there is something happening that you disagree with, you must find a way to stop it.

As dentists, a critical part of what we do includes getting the whole family involved in oral health care for these children, including any of the kids' babysitters or caretakers. These aren't rules that are only applied at home. These aren't rules that are only applied at school. You know the rules, and your job is to enforce them. The kids only get chocolate milk once a week, not once a week and also whenever Grandma or his aunt feeds them. We try to hold our kids and their parents to these rules.

The sooner we can spread the message to the parents about sugar (in liquid drinks) leading to tooth decay, the better. Tooth decay will open up a whole other box that will force us to talk about pediatric dentistry. When we see kids under the age of three years old with developed cavities from milk, apple juice, or chocolate milk, the subject of the conversation becomes treatment rather than prevention. We cannot leave cavities or decay in primary teeth and baby teeth.

The Importance Of Baby Teeth

Parents hold common misconceptions about baby teeth. "Why does my child need to worry about his baby teeth? They're just going to fall out, aren't they?" Here's the problem with that. Baby teeth are serving two major functions for children: retaining space for adult teeth and developing speech habits.

- Number One, baby teeth hold positions and space for the adult teeth that will come in later. Think of baby teeth as mini-retainers for your kids. The baby tooth is there. It starts getting wiggly once the adult tooth begins growing up underneath it. The adult tooth pushes through, and the baby tooth falls out. The adult tooth has now taken its proper spot in the mouth. If the baby tooth gets a giant cavity or breaks, and it has to be pulled out a year or two years early, that adult tooth loses its guide. It can grow in crooked. It can grow behind another tooth, in front of the mouth. So, really, that baby tooth plays an important role in the positioning of teeth through adolescence.
- Number Two, the two front teeth help children develop speech patterns for their adult life, and the lack of front teeth can keep children from being able to speak clearly. Bedtime milk creates cavities in the two front teeth. If those teeth get decayed beyond repair and must be pulled out early, we have noticed that children develop speech impediments. They have difficulty learning speech and they're delayed in their speech development. Those front teeth are so important for many of the sounds we make: the "S" sound, the "Th" sound, etc. At three or four years old, kids are working at developing and fine-tuning their

speech patterns; they're learning how to communicate. If they have missing teeth, they will get saddled with another disadvantage—the inability to speak clearly and effectively to other kids. By getting rid of those decayed teeth too early, they're developing bad speech habits that are hard to break later in life.

These are things we tell parents regarding the importance of baby teeth. When talking to parents about why baby teeth are important, we can't just say, "They're going to fall out later, anyway. Let's just pull them out. There are other teeth coming in." Those little teeth serve a crucial purpose.

Pediatric Dentists

What happens when decay appears in the teeth? Now, we're going to bring up the pediatric dentist. Since most general dentists aren't necessarily equipped to work on children, there's a special dentistry field called pediatric dentistry. A pediatric dentist knows how to handle the behavior management of a child. This includes the behavior of an anxious child or a nervous child. Pediatric dentists are specially trained and equipped to handle the problems unique to little patients.

A pediatric dentist does the same thing that we do—takes some extra steps in preparing to treat children. It can be as simple as just talking them through procedures. They can use a little bit of nitrous oxide, commonly known as "laughing gas," to ease the anxiety. Alternatively, they can use sedation, which means that the pediatric dentist will put your children to sleep to work on them.

I tell parents (and the pediatric dentists will say the same thing) that putting your child to sleep is always the last option. It's never the first option. General anesthesia is something that should be avoided in children when at all possible. It should just be the fallback alternative. You should never say, "Just put them to sleep to get the work done." There are many adverse side effects to general anesthesia in children, things that we really want to avoid.

The Dental Timeline

I've focused on the "gap" in dentistry—the part of the population of patients who really aren't discussed much—and the timing of their dental visits. Young patients, from the day of birth to about two years old, are the forgotten patients. Pediatricians don't really have a strong enough grasp on the dental needs of children, or they don't clearly convey the importance of dental care for that age.

A child's first dental check-up should come at 18 months of age. Traditionally, that's the first time when general and pediatric dentists are comfortable with doing routine check-ups. Of course, the caveat is that if there's any trauma—accidents, or any other reasons for your child to come earlier—then certainly bring them in. In terms of routine check-ups, we like to start them at 18 months of age. I always tell the parents that those visits really aren't for the child; they are meant for the parents. The value of this appointment goes far beyond whatever we can do in the chair. There are many things we review in this visit, mostly regarding good tooth care habit formation and diet.

At this point, we expect that pacifiers should be gone. This goes hand-in-glove with the habit formation process; at 18 months of age, children should be done with their pacifiers and their bottles. ("Bottle" also means anything with a nipple that they like to feed on; if they're being breastfed, we like for them to start getting weaned.) If they have not given these up, it's time to begin the process, because continually sucking on pacifiers or bottles or fingers is actually causing skeletal change. They're developing the dreaded overbite, the bucktoothed look that parents always worry about. This is a developmental stage.

Many parents will say, "It's genetic. I had it. My mother had it." While it can be genetic, it's usually habit-based. Thumb sucking, pacifier sucking, bottle sucking—any one of those habits needs to get curbed before 18 months of age. If we fail to accomplish this, it will actually pull the front jaw forward—that comes from sucking and can cause problems for the orthodontist later. Usually at 18 months, a lot of our little patients still have pacifiers and bottles, and we start telling parents the news: "Hey, we're going to cut that back."

When the pacifier and the bottle are removed, a lot of children will resort to finding something else to suck on, usually their thumb or their fingers. It's a lot harder to break the habit of a kid's thumb or finger than a pacifier or bottle. The parents must get involved there and make sure that it's a firm "No"; that habit must be broken right from the beginning. Kids cannot be allowed to put thumbs or fingers into their mouths. Many kids will do that for soothing purposes, but at 18 months, they're old enough to be trained to stop it. They can be allowed to self-soothe in other ways (a stuffed animal, music, or rocking motions), but the first and foremost priority is to get those things solved for the child and get those fingers out of the mouth—whatever it takes.

The second item that we review at these 18-month check-ups deals with diet; it means getting rid of milk during the bedtime routine. The first question I ask the parents at this stage is, "Explain your bedtime routine." Often, we hear this list: "We give our son or daughter a bath. We read them a book. We give them a bottle of milk. Then we put them to bed." I tell all the parents,

"Wrong answer." Milk must be eliminated from the bedtime routine at this age. Milk during the day or at dinnertime is fine, but once we start going into the nighttime routine, water must be substituted. Milk contains lots of natural sugars. Putting a kid to sleep who's just had a drink of milk will start the first onset of tooth decay and cavities, whether it's given to them in a bottle or a cup. As dentists, we see it all the time. I always tell parents, "*Milk cannot be the last drink your child has before bed time.* That needs to be water and we need to start brushing as part of the bedtime routine as well."

We hear this comment over and over: "My child doesn't let me brush his teeth." My response is, "You have to win that battle." This isn't a negotiable point. They have to start getting used to brushing teeth at an early age, in order to establish a good habit for their future. Yes, they will fight you the first five times or so, just like they fought you the first five times you wanted to get them to take a nap or a shower or anything else. It's a fight, but you'll win it. You just have to get through it.

First Check-Up—18 Months

At that first 18-month check-up, for most parents, we focus on these issues: bedtime brushing, water at bedtime, and getting rid of the pacifier and bottle. If that first visit doesn't happen until 24 or 36 months, if those habits have not been broken by the time that the child is three years old, then we start seeing irreversible damage. We see widespread tooth decay, skeletal changes with overbites and buck teeth; each one of these three things will absolutely lead to a long-term installment of orthodontic braces. Those consequences are things that we can predict when we see children in this situation.

Also, at the first check-up, parents usually learn more than the kids do. However, it's good to have your child there as an introduction. "This is the dentist. I'm sitting on a chair on Mom or Dad's lap. They're going to put some stuff in my mouth. Okay." Again, they're going to cry at that visit, just like when a pediatrician gives a vaccine to your child. Just because there will be tears doesn't mean you should be embarrassed or wait until later to bring in your child. After the first 18-month visit, we always recommend that children come for their check-ups every six months.

24 Months

By 18 to 24 months, kids really should have developed all of the teeth in their mouth, and their dentist can watch the molars coming in. By 24 months, the dentist will have an idea if there are any congenitally missing teeth or dental abnormalities. The second check-up, which we do at 24 months, will be focused on your child's development and his teeth. Also, I tell parents, "It's time to grade your homework from the 18-month check-up. Are we off the pacifier? Are we off the bottle? Describe your bedtime routine." Almost always, the parents have heeded most of the advice, and we start to see really good healthy, positive check-ups from this point forward.

If you and your child have somehow managed to miss the salient points from the 18-month visit, it will begin to reveal itself in your child's mouth by 24 months. Now there may be the need to actually work in the mouth. This is when we bring in the laughing gas—nitrous oxide.

Laughing gas is an extremely safe alternative that eliminates any tension or anxiety. It basically involves your child breathing in a little air that causes them to get a little loopy. The dentist does the work and, as soon as that mask comes off, the child snaps back in a couple of seconds. They might be dizzy for a minute, but there's no long-lasting effect and no grogginess because the child is never out. They're breathing on their own the whole time. They're responsive. For us, nitrous oxide is by far the preferred method of treating pediatric patients whenever possible.

Finally, if you do have a child with extensive decay or a child with such high anxiety that it's not possible to treat them in any manner, then, unfortunately, there are times when we do have to start using dental anesthesia. When we have conversations with parents about their kid's level of decay, we always hope that we can treat him under laughing gas and not have to resort to general anesthesia. Most of the time, though, all of this hassle could have been prevented; most of the time, it's diet-related. It's such a simple fix!

30 to 36 Months

During the time frame of 30 to 36 months of age, most pediatric and general dentists (including my office) will start taking X-rays on children. We don't normally take them earlier because we're just waiting for the baby teeth to erupt, to emerge in the mouth. By 36 months, all of the baby teeth should have arrived. At 36 months, we can take X-rays and see cavities at a really small stage before they're big enough to be seen otherwise. We can start working on very small cavities really early to avoid more damage.

Early Childhood

With good X-rays, we can also make sure that the first of the underlying adult teeth are also being developed in the proper location, that they will arrive on schedule, and we'll be able to see them develop over time. We can see them forming and moving in as the baby teeth get smaller and smaller. The first set of adult teeth will grow in at six years old; we refer to them as "first molars" or "six-year-old molars." They will come in at the back of the mouth—one on the top left, one on the top right, one on the bottom left, and one on the bottom right. These teeth, unfortunately, are the most likely teeth for developing cavities in a child's mouth; you will keep those teeth from six years old (hopefully) until you're 96 years old. Those teeth don't go anywhere. They are permanent teeth.

Between six and seven years of age, the front baby teeth will fall out and the permanent incisors will come in, four at the top and four at the bottom. Eight adult teeth will be growing in there as well. Also, those are the teeth that will be there forever. Between the ages of five-and-a-half and six-and-half, it's more important than ever to actually follow through with dental check-ups—this is when brushing has to be very, very good. To be successful, this involves child brushing and parent brushing, or the parent watching the child brushing. If boundaries have been established with a healthy diet and healthy liquid diets at younger ages, we won't start seeing cavities on these back molars because the sugar content is under control.

In our office, we see our kids get through their baby teeth stage cavity-free—the brushing habit has been good, and the diet is under control. Those kids are far less likely to get cavities through their teenage years. Most of that success can be credited to good diet. It's a pivotal part in tooth development and tooth formation. The key is really a healthy and a low-sugar diet; we need to get that message to the parents. That's the key focus in our practice.

The Importance Of Sealants

Sealants play a role in preventive dentistry along with diet. These are some of the first questions that parents will often ask: "What's the best way I can prevent my kids from getting cavities? What do I do to make sure my kids have healthy teeth?" We'll harp on diet and brushing, but that's when your dentist can intervene and help out with dental sealants. The way we describe sealant to the six-year-old or the parent is that it's almost like a clear nail polish that will go over the top or the biting surface of the tooth; it will prevent any sugar or sticky stuff from sticking, therefore preventing cavity growth on top of the teeth. Sealants are placed very non-invasively. It's basically just a small resin that fills in the grooves of the tooth. It almost makes your tooth feel glassy, like an ice skating rink, so you feel like nothing will stick on that tooth. Sealants are an incredible way to prevent cavities on the chewing and biting surfaces of these adult molars. They are probably a dentist's best tool in terms of preventing cavities. However, they do not prevent cavities on the side of the teeth, and liquids can coat the sides of the teeth, so this is when we start talking about the dreaded sugary drinks again.

At this point, we start worrying about decay in between the teeth, which brings up the next step: "When should my kid begin flossing?" My answer is, "Any time that you can get them to start is great." By six years old, it needs to be mandatory—at least once or twice a week. We don't really expect six-year-olds to have the best manual dexterity to floss themselves, but parent intervention is great, and parents should still help their children with this step. Besides avoiding sugary drinks and regularly brushing, flossing is the best way to prevent cavities on these molars between the teeth. Just moving floss between the teeth will help break up anything that's stuck on the teeth, remove any sugars, and will go a long way toward preventing decay from forming on the sides of the teeth.

So, at six years old or whenever those first molars grow in, we traditionally recommend sealants as soon as possible. Every kid is different. Every kid will develop at a different pace. With growth, they tend to get their molars at an earlier stage. It's not uncommon to see girls with molars at five to five-and-a-half years old. On the flip side, boys will develop a little slower at this age, so it may not be uncommon to see a boy at six-and-a-half or seven before he gets his first molars.

The next set of adult teeth to come in will be their pre-molars at nine and 10 years old. These are the teeth that grow in in front of the molars. Again, we put sealants on those teeth as well. All of the same rules apply to that first molar as to those pre-molars: sealants, flossing, reduce sugary drinks.

At 12 years old, the second molars have usually grown behind the six-year-old molars. The second set, the 12-year-old molars, will also get sealants at that visit. Finally, after age six and 12, the 18-year-old molars come in, more commonly known as wisdom teeth. These teeth generally do not get sealants placed on them for a variety of reasons. First of all, they tend not to grow in straight. Most of the time, they'll get impacted or they'll be extracted. In rare cases, the child shows up at age 18 with perfectly straight wisdom teeth and there's room in the mouth, so we can place sealants on them. But, more often than not, they don't get sealed because of one of the issues we talked about—either they don't grow in straight, they get taken out, or they get removed for a variety of reasons.

By the age of 12, all of the adult teeth that will ever get sealants have arrived, and everything has been sealed by then. Those six-year-old, nine-year-old, and twelve-year-old visits are big preventive visits for our sealants. If applied correctly and maintained well, sealants should last many, many years. Parents ask, "Do they get sealants every year?" The answer is no. Sealants should last between three and five years, and sometimes they can last even longer. Ask your dentist if a sealant does pop up on a tooth, because many times they can just re-apply a sealant at the next visit. If the child gets a six-year-old sealant, usually it won't need to get resealed. Around the age of 12, if someone notices that the sealant is wearing out or the sealant has fallen off, the teeth can get resealed.

Dental Requirements For School Children

Often, parents don't bring their children to a dentist until something goes wrong. We asked a parent who brought in a seven-year-old, "When was the last time that he saw a dentist?" Answer: "Nothing's ever bothered him." I think that's never the right answer. When we took an X-ray, the kid had three cavities and we needed to do a root canal. In many of our offices, we started having to treat these children on an emergency basis during school hours; we were writing out tremendous numbers of school notes. Kids would arrive with an infection, cracked teeth, or they would need a root canal.

One of our accomplishments has come out of our visits to the public school systems in some of these cities where our offices are located. We've asked them, "As far as vaccinations and such, what are the yearly requirements for their medical and dental exams?" The answer is always the same: "Well, they need a vaccine record and a physical." We ask about dentistry and they look a little surprised. "No, there's nothing in place for that." Why are there no requirements for dental screening?

We've made a big move toward getting dental exams to be mandatory for school children in public schools before each year starts. We've enacted a program called "Summer Smiles"; we want children to get check-ups in the summer when it doesn't interfere with school hours. Let's prevent and diagnose things that could become problems later on. Let's get them scheduled on the weekends or after school. Let's get the work done with parents understanding what's going on in their child's mouth, not waiting until something hurts so that the child has to miss a day or two of school to fix a dental problem.

Part of that push has been going to the public schools and trying to get schools on a local basis to encourage parents to bring their kids to check-ups, to make them mandatory. We've even gone through a lot of state-funded day care centers in these cities and offered our services for free. "Hey, every year, call us in whenever you want. We'll do a check-up on all these kids again, right in your house; if they are eighteen months, 24 months, 30 months old, bring them. We will come back every year."

We do routine screenings on all of them. We write a letter home to Mom and Dad. "Calvin looks good. You can still bring him in." On the other hand, "We see some things we don't like. If you don't have a dentist, please come to see us."

There's a great reach that we can have if we can get into the school systems. It's my dream that the state of New Jersey will follow what a few other states have done, which is mandating their public school systems to have regular dental check-ups, whether it's every year or every two years. There should be at least something every year so that kids are being looked at and their dental health is being treated the same as the rest of their health. Like I said, it's also our goal to make this a national movement. If we can at least get started in New Jersey, it will go a long way toward helping us accomplish what we need to accomplish, in terms of keeping our kids' oral health at a good state—above all, keeping our kids healthy.

(This content should be used for informational purposes only. It does not create a doctor-patient relationship with any reader and should not be construed as medical advice. If you need medical advice, please contact a doctor in your community who can assess the specifics of your situation.)

4

Complete Health Dentistry: Considering How Dental Care Affects a Patient's Overall Health

by Steven Gusfa, D.D.S.

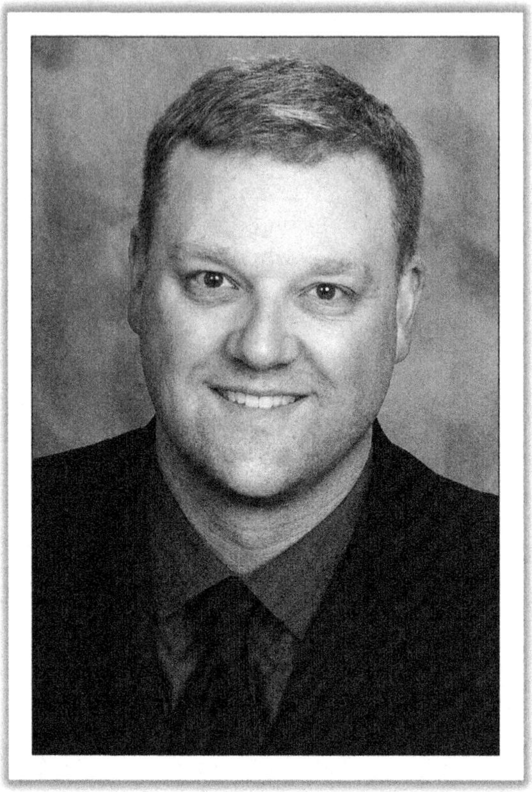

Steven Gusfa, D.D.S.
Gusfa Dental Clinic
Dearborn, Michigan
www.gusfadentalclinic.com

Dr. Steven Gusfa graduated from the University of Michigan School of Dentistry in 2001. He has 14 years of experience practicing dentistry. His Professional Memberships include: American Dental Association 2001 to present, Michigan Dental, Association 2001 to present, Detroit District Dental Society (Southwestern Branch) 2001 to present. He has been active within these organizations as Secretary of Southwestern Branch

2004 to 2006, President of Southwestern Branch 2006 to 2008, Secretary of Detroit District Dental Society 2008 to 2009, Vice President of Detroit District Dental Society 2009 to 2010, President Elect of Detroit District Dental Society 2010 to 2011, President Detroit District Dental Society 2011 to 2012 and MDA House of Delegates 2005 to 2013. Dr. Gusfa was also inducted into the Pierre Fauchard Academy in 2007, the International College of Dentists in 2011, received the Detroit District Dental Society's New Dentist of the Year Award in 2005, and the Michigan Dental Association's Matt Uday New Dentist Leadership Award in 2011.

In his free time Dr. Gusfa enjoys spending time with his family, especially his two children who are his raison d'être. He also enjoys the outdoors, attending sporting events, cooking great barbecue, and tweaking his almost perfect signature BBQ sauce.

Complete Health Dentistry: Considering How Dental Care Affects a Patient's Overall Health

My Personal Story and Journey

Growing up in Plymouth, Michigan, I had a wonderful childhood. My parents had a strong faith that they instilled in their children, and family life was very important. I had an older sister and a younger sister. My younger sister was quite special to us—she had Down syndrome. Growing up alongside a sibling with Down syndrome made everything a little bit different—it was the event that had the greatest influence on my life. It really put things into perspective. I learned what was truly important in life and that simple accomplishments can be viewed as significantly different through another person's eyes. Celebrating all of the little things and daily small miracles was very important and well worth the effort.

My younger sister passed in 1991 when I was 15 years old. Everything was a struggle for her, but watching her consistent approach to everything was amazing. She never shied away from anything, no matter how difficult the challenge. Every day she had the same attitude: unconditional love for everyone around her. She touched everyone around her in a very special way. There was nothing you could do to irritate her. It was amazing to see that in somebody. I mean everyone has some faults or bad days, but my sister never wavered from loving everyone around her. It was beyond amazing, and I was privileged to be a part of her life. There were what seemed to be 5,000 people at her funeral, and she was only 12 years old when she passed.

My parents were also amazing people with a strong faith that they passed on to each of their children. You would assume that my sister's condition and death would have rattled their faith, but it did not; it strengthened their faith. That gave me a sense of comfort. Watching my sister go through death and watching how my parents handled that experience removed the fear of death for me. In the moments right after her passing, knowing that she was still around made me believe in the after-life.

I have had experiences after my sister passed when I knew she was with me. One moment in particular was probably about a year after she had gone and I was having a bad day. You never forget and you never truly get over the loss, you just learn to live with it. As I was walking down the stairway in our childhood home, I accidentally knocked her picture off the wall and it tumbled down the stairs. Nothing happened to the photo or the picture frame, but when it hit the bottom of the stairs, the alarm clock in her room went off. I went up to her room to turn it off. By the time I got in there, it had already stopped. It was then that I noticed the alarm clock was not plugged in. It wasn't really an eerie moment for me, and I was not scared or freaked out. It was a very happy moment because I felt comforted. There are times when I remember something and a kind of rush, a tingly feeling, comes over me; I know she is in the room with me. Because of the experience of losing my sister, I am not afraid of what may come or even of the death process. I am concerned, if I am taken early, that my children will have to live without me; but I know that I can be there with them and it relieves some of that fear. My sister's unconditional love, her passing, and my children have made my faith extremely strong.

If just one person reads about my experience and God chooses to open their eyes, then I am blessed to be a part of the process of God working in another person's life, bringing them to faith in Christ. That is a huge event in anyone's life. The passing of my sister and the experience of the birth of my children confirmed my faith. I cannot understand how a parent who has experienced the birth of a child cannot believe in God. I cannot imagine receiving a gift like that and not wondering where it came from.

I chose to become a dentist for a number of different reasons, including my second-hand experience of dentistry. My father was a dentist. I had the opportunity to watch him daily, and seeing how much he enjoyed his patients and his work was a tremendous experience. It was the first taste of dentistry that I had as a child. I attended Detroit Catholic Central High School before going on to Kalamazoo College. At the beginning of my undergraduate studies, I did not intend to become a dentist. However, after exploring my options over time, I remembered the life that my dad had experienced while I was growing up and all that the profession gave to him, and I decided that dentistry was a good fit for me as well. After making a decision in my junior year of college and after graduation from Kalamazoo College, I attended dental school at the University of Michigan. I have never looked back since that junior year decision.

Dentistry is a noble profession. It allows you to lead a good life, go home to your family each evening and stay at home with your family, unlike in some other medical professions. That is what I do and I love every day of it. I am married with two children—a six-year-old daughter and a three-year-old son. Both are great ages, and I enjoy every moment that I have with them. I love watching them grow up and I look forward to a good future for them.

As an adult, the three biggest influential events in my life were my wedding day and the birth of each of my children. Pledging my life to my wife, and having a companion who is wonderful and beautiful, provides me with comfort and joy. We enjoy doing things together and enjoy raising our kids together. Hopefully, we can provide them with the same quality of childhood that we both had while growing up. My children give me something to work for each day. Making sure that I provide for their needs today and in the future drives me to do my best each day.

My Philosophy Of Dentistry

My philosophy of dentistry is to provide complete health dentistry in my office. This means making sure that we consider everything we do in the sense of how it relates to or affects the entire body and the patient's overall health. I work from a preventive model. I am concerned about my patients' oral health as well as their overall health and wellness.

Where Do I See Dentistry Going?

Technological advancements seem limitless at this point. That is one important part of the future of dentistry. Almost anything that you can dream about may eventually happen. I never thought that people would have the ability to regrow teeth, which seems to be around the corner. The other part of dentistry's future, at some point, will be standing side-by-side with the medical profession from an overall health standpoint. Dentistry has always somewhat taken a backseat in the medical profession, but we are gaining ground. It should be a partnership. The screenings and advantages that we can provide to patients can be quite advantageous to the overall health of our country. I see us standing alongside medicine and achieving the goal of better health for our patients.

As dentists, we sometimes see our patients more frequently than their medical doctors see them. Whether checking blood pressure or looking for oral signs of systemic disease, dentists can save peoples' lives by playing a role in prevention and early detection. Enhancing someone's smile can do several things from a personal and a wellness standpoint. Changing a person's smile may result in that person getting that dream job or giving that person the confidence to go out and find a spouse. Changing a smile not only enhances a person's beauty, it also gives that person a lot of confidence.

I am already experiencing more cooperation from the medical profession than in the past. Patients have been referred to me prior to their replacement surgeries to ensure that they get oral clearance before surgery. One of my patients was in the process of undergoing cancer therapy that included chemo and radiation treatment. The primary care doctor wanted to make sure that there were no teeth in any condition that would prevent the patient from continuing with the treatment, and no teeth that might create an emergency. This alignment of medical treatment is happening slower than I think it should, but it is beginning to happen. However, I am fairly proactive. I will directly call a doctor when I have concerns about one of my patients, or in the case of a patient who would benefit from tooth repair before having other medical treatment.

Other doctors don't always understand the amount of inflammation that can occur in someone's mouth. Sometimes it is difficult to get an audience with them. Sometimes they have an attitude of already knowing what a dentist will say, but they do not. Many doctors are open-minded, and protocols are changing, but many are still hesitant. I think that the American Dental Association, and even our local Michigan Dental Association, has done a wonderful job educating the public and doctors about the relationship between overall health and oral systemic disease. The wheels are turning. In 10 years, I think it will be a completely different environment.

As dentists, we are moving further away from being problem-fixers than when I first began practicing. Rather than the patient coming in with a chief complaint, or dentists simply addressing a chief complaint, we are taking a more proactive approach to prevention. We want to avoid any issues and provide care that sets the patient on a road to being healthy forever, rather than dealing with things only after they break down. Even during my stint in dental school, the patient exams were structured from the standpoint of starting with a chief complaint and working forward from there. I have moved away from that model of dentistry. Now, I perform a comprehensive exam before I ask about what may be bothering a patient or what may have brought the patient to my office. Many times, building a comprehensive picture to view the situation as a whole rather than in bits and pieces has an impact on the treatment that we provide.

Another change during my lifetime as a dentist is that we are now able to restore someone's oral health back to a point in time when the person had better oral health, such as when they were younger. Dentistry is the one branch of the medical field that can truly restore someone's teeth to the way they were in their teen years, through implants and cosmetic dentistry. Technological advances have come a long way toward making people's teeth "brand new" again.

Preventive Dentistry And Its Importance

Earlier, I discussed taking a more proactive approach to prevent oral systemic disease, which is part of preventive dentistry. The other part of preventive dentistry is educating patients about the best homecare practices. In my office, my recommendation is to brush three to four times a day, floss at least once a day, and use a mouth rinse at least twice a day. We couple that with nutrition counseling to make sure that patients have a good, healthy, balanced diet. If they are consuming foods that can cause oral disease, most commonly foods with sugars, then they should be made aware that prolonged exposure to those sugars is detrimental. They need to be conscious of when they are consuming them and what is happening after. For example, having a glass of orange juice right before bedtime seems benign; however, it can create havoc if you do not brush your teeth afterwards and let the orange juice sit in your mouth all night. That can create all sorts of big problems later on.

Addressing things early on, before inflammation comes into play, can prevent much more serious conditions. Another proactivity example is addressing a simple crack before the tooth breaks. Dentists work hard to identify any clinical signs of systemic disease, such as anemia and hypothyroidism. There is a laundry list of about 300 things that we can look for when treating a patient. For example, a complaint of "burning mouth syndrome" is a common symptom for vitamin deficiencies and anemia. If we identify something that is a symptom of another condition, we advise that patient to consult with his or her physicians for blood work and an exam. We also follow up on that with the patient. In my opinion, preventive dentistry is taking a proactive approach to overall health as well as oral health.

People often ask this question: "Can I afford it?" In a preventive world, the question should be, "Can you afford not to do it?" Whenever an exam or a procedure is delayed or you avoid treatment, it always ends up being more expensive in the end. When you are thinking about how your current smile may be affecting your career or your home life, in my opinion, the expense of delaying or ignoring treatment far outweighs the expense or the fee involved with the treatment. There are many different ways to make dental treatment more affordable. You can discuss a payment plan with your dentist, use CareCredit, or explore other options.

Statistics often shed a bright light on why we cannot afford to NOT take care of our oral health. Recent reports suggest one out of every two heart attacks in the United States gets triggered by gum disease—not necessarily caused, but triggered. Fifty to eighty percent of the American population has gum disease. People with gum disease are twice as likely to die from heart disease and three times more likely to die from stroke. Diabetes coupled with bleeding gums increases a patient's risk of premature death by 400 to 700 percent. Pregnant women with gum disease have only a one in seven chance of giving birth to a healthy child.

Every time you breathe in, you are aspirating some of the bacteria in your mouth. Every time you swallow, you are swallowing some of those bacteria. Bacteria in your mouth can travel all over your body through your blood stream. Those bacteria can cause heart disease, high blood pressure, and stroke. Bacteria will also increase your risk for a long list of other diseases, such as arthritis, pancreatic cancer, and kidney cancer.

The Importance Of An Attractive Smile

This is another piece of the wellness puzzle. It is important because it can play a big role in a person's mental health. Many of my patients tell me that they do not want to smile because of the look of their teeth. What is that doing for them from a mental health standpoint? Smiling is important. Laughing is important. If you are consciously avoiding those situations, it may have a big impact on your well-being.

Again, an attractive smile can put you on the frontline for a job or for meeting your significant other. It can help you gain respect. If you are speaking with another human being, you do not want them constantly looking at your teeth and wondering why you are not taking care of your teeth rather than paying attention to what you are saying; even worse, you don't want them discounting what you are saying. Therefore, it is very important for your overall well-being that you maintain an attractive, healthy smile.

What Is The Cost Of A Smile Makeover?

There are solutions for everyone at every level of investment. We can always find something to enhance a person's smile that fits into any budget or lifestyle. It may be veneers, Invisalign® treatment, cosmetic bonding, or a combination of several procedures. We also have temporary solutions that literally snap on to your teeth; they can last up to a year or two. They are good for patients with a limited income who have an immediate need to improve their smile (for an upcoming wedding or other event) and they do not want to make a huge investment. There is always something that we can do, regardless of a person's budget.

For gummy smiles, there are some great new techniques. I have just been reading and hearing about these solutions for the last couple of months. The procedure is called LipStaT™. In the past, the only solutions for gummy smiles were surgery or BOTOX® injections every three months. Now, a simple surgical procedure that takes half an hour can change the position of the lip permanently. It heals within two weeks. There is no discomfort involved that cannot be controlled by Motrin® for a few days following the procedure. It can enhance the lip line or change how the lip line interacts with the teeth. It also affects how the lip appears because of muscles that are always tugging, pulling, and curling back under. We can do something very simple to relieve that and make the lip lay flatter against the teeth in a more ideal position. Cosmetic dentistry is always improving and there are solutions and options for every person.

How Does Fluoride Help Prevent Tooth Decay?

There are three ways that fluoride helps prevent tooth decay. Before we get to the three ways, it would be best to preface that discussion with an explanation of how tooth decay occurs.

Basically, it is a teeter-tottering effect between the bacteria and the tooth. When bacteria form plaque around the teeth and start consuming the sugars and other food debris in our mouth, the result is the production of acid. The acid dissolves the calcium and phosphate minerals on the surface of the enamel on the tooth. That process is called demineralization. When it has pierced through the enamel, a cavity is created. Sometimes the acid in the plaque can be neutralized on the enamel surface and the process can be reversed through remineralization.

Fluoride disrupts the teeter-tottering between demineralization and remineralization, and tips the process towards remineralization in three ways. First, the fluoride that we incorporate during tooth development (when we are young), through the structure that develops the enamel, makes the teeth more resistant to the acid effect. The other two ways that fluoride plays a key role occurs after the development of the teeth, from the consistent exposure of our teeth and the plaque to fluoride, whether it is in the form of toothpaste or varnishes.

The presence of low levels of fluoride in the plaque and saliva encourage remineralization, ensuring an improved quality of the enamel crystals that are laid down. Fluoride also reduces the ability of the plaque to produce acid. Of course, the most common way to apply fluoride is through the daily use of toothpaste. However, an even stronger way of utilizing fluoride is to apply a varnish at regular dental health check-up visits, which is like putting a protective coating on the teeth. I recommend this for patients of all ages. The American Dental Association also recommends this procedure for patients of all ages. Varnishing becomes an even more powerful tool when patients reach their senior years; dentists are beginning to see increased incidents of cavities forming on root surfaces that are exposed over time.

Utilizing fluoride in those situations can be very beneficial to the patient in reducing the risk of tooth decay.

Dental Implants: The Closest Choice To A Natural Tooth

In my opinion, when a tooth must be replaced, dental implants are about the closest possible option to a natural tooth. The implanted teeth are fixed. They stand alone. They do not place extra stress on any of the neighboring teeth. Dental implants are made out of titanium; many times, they end up being the strongest teeth in the mouth. The success rate is outstanding. In fact, I think that dental implants have the best success rate of any procedure that we do in dentistry—about 98 percent or better. Dental implants have the best chance of lasting for the rest of our lives, whereas none of the other alternatives have that ability.

Alternatives to dental implants, such as bridges and partial dentures, have limited life spans. In both cases, these alternatives can put excess stress on the neighboring teeth to which they are anchored, causing other problems. Bridges, when they fail, can actually take out one of the neighboring teeth with them. In my opinion, the best solution for replacing a tooth is a dental implant. It is a relatively easy process and quite comfortable in comparison to some of the other options. It is much easier than having a tooth removed.

Are Electric Toothbrushes Worth The Cost?

In my opinion, they are definitely worth the cost. It takes the work out of a lot of the technique involved with brushing teeth. We always recommend that our patients make circles with their toothbrushes, and brush each of the four corners for about 30 seconds at a time, without pressing too hard.

Some of the newer brushes do all of this for us, including the circular motions. We just need to hold the brush in the right place. Some of them will even time the contact with the teeth, and tell you when to move on to the next area. The newer toothbrushes can connect to your mobile telephone and submit reports to your dentist as to whether or not you have been brushing correctly. This makes it easy for us to follow up with our patients to see whether or not they are taking our recommendations. Technology has come a long way in those areas. I definitely recommend electric toothbrushes to all my patients.

The Problem Of Bad Breath

More often than not, the most common cause of bad breath is the proliferation of bacteria on a patient's tongue. Most people do not brush their tongue regularly; this is the leading cause of bad breath. In those situations, we prescribe a tongue scraper. We can also take it a step further if that simple "debridement" (i.e., scraping) of the tongue does not work.

We can also discuss different types of mouth rinses with our patients. Most patients incorrectly use mouth rinses. Most commonly, patients use them only once a day, even though 90% of the mouth rinses on the market are only effective if they are used twice a day. If mouth rinses do not work, it's possible to take the process to the next step by adjusting the levels of certain bacteria in the mouth through prescribing a simple antibiotic that targets the bacteria. In effect, this resets the balance of bacteria. The patient takes it twice a day for two weeks. It can have a significant effect on the balance of bacteria by reducing the harmful odor-creating bacteria that is causing bad breath.

Bleeding Gums: Signs Of Bigger Problems

When people ask me what they should do if their gums bleed when they brush their teeth, I ask them what they would do if every time they brushed their hair their scalp bled. You would have your scalp checked out by a professional.

Bleeding gums should definitely be a point of concern because bleeding is a sign of a serious inflammation. The surface of the inside of our mouth is similar to the surface on the palm of our hand. If your mouth bleeds or your gums bleed when you are brushing your teeth, it is analogous to having an open wound on your hand. If you had an open wound on your hand, you would not think that was okay—you would seek medical attention. The same thing is true with your mouth. Having an open wound of that size, a wound that is not healing, is a big concern. Most of the time, the problem of bleeding gums is related to periodontal disease.

Handling Dental Emergencies

Time is always of the essence in dental emergencies. Cell phone technology is a huge advantage that can benefit the patient. I take emergency calls at any time. My emergency phone number is available to all my patients. My patients call for a variety of different reasons. For those with a cell phone, they can snap a picture of the problem so that I can view the issue remotely. By viewing the problem remotely, I am able to specifically address the emergency to determine whether it is something that needs to be handled right away or if it can wait until the next day. If the problem needs to be addressed immediately, I meet them at the office. In the case of a dental emergency, I advise anyone to make sure that you will be able to reach your dentist; keep your cell phone handy to take a photo to send to your dentist.

This is especially true for children. The parents at my dentistry practice get overly concerned about many things just like I do with my children, and they are often not sure about whether the problem is an emergency or not. I tell them to take a quick photo of the problem area so that I can take a look. It works out really well. Many times, a child will knock a few teeth on the table, or something like that, and the affected area looks a lot worse than it is. Most of the time, I can tell a lot by a picture. I can either have the parents bring the child to the office, if it is truly an emergency, or calm them down so they are not worrying through the night or over the weekend until they can come into the office during normal business hours.

Dental Disease And Treatments

Periodontal disease is a chronic bacterial infection of the mouth. It causes a breakdown in the support structure around the teeth. Bacteria start to build up around the teeth and the gum line, and the gums begin to pull away from the teeth. There is a simple explanation for what happens. Bacteria can get down in between the gums and cause the bone to break down around the tooth. It is a very dangerous disease because it is typically associated with absolutely no symptoms until the teeth become extremely loose. Several contributors do come into play when assessing a person's chances of developing periodontal disease: genetics, diet, home care, systemic diseases (such as diabetes), and tobacco use. These can all contribute to periodontal disease.

Many times, we can treat periodontal disease in a non-invasive way with gum therapy. I like to call this treatment "gum therapy" rather than using the technical term of "scaling and root planing." In our office, we offer gum therapy followed up with antibiotics which specifically target the bacteria that are causing trouble. If that does not work, the patient may need to visit a specialist. However, I do not like to talk about that option unless it is absolutely necessary, since it is not a pleasant experience.

Regarding specialists, my philosophy is this: if a specialist can provide higher quality care for one of my patients and do the necessary procedure better than I can, I want that patient to go to the specialist. If gum therapy does not work, if something else needs to be done that I do not regularly do, a periodontist may be in order. If it is a challenging tooth with a challenging anatomy, I would rather have a specialist handle the procedure for my patient, knowing that the specialist will provide a much higher quality of care than I can. I treat each of my patients as if they are family. If I would not do a procedure on my sister or my mom, I would not do it on any of my other patients.

What Is A Root Canal?

A root canal is one procedure that I will refer to a specialist. If there is an infection within the root itself, involving the nerve tissue and blood supply of the tooth, the best way to remove that infection is to hollow out the tooth using a series of files and then seal the root with a rubbery material (called gutta-percha) to seal it from the inside out. The roots of our teeth do not typically handle infection very well. For example, if there is an infection in the ear, many times the body can take care of itself. If there is an infection within the tooth, it is something that the body cannot deal with on its own.

Temporarily, the infection can be treated with an antibiotic, though in most cases, the infection will come back. When it comes back, it is usually worse. The body is not very good at clearing infection out from the inside of the tooth. There is really no alternative other than a root canal, unless you want to have the tooth removed.

The typical way to handle infection in the root of a tooth is from the top down, such as a root canal. That is the most predictable way to handle the infection. In some instances, if this has not been a successful method, another procedure, called an apicoectomy, can be performed to reseal the other end under the root. This is typically a last resort if the traditional way does not work. When the specialist begins resealing the end of the root, he has to remove some of the root. Since this makes the root shorter and disrupts the support of the tooth, it is not done very often.

After a root canal, the tooth is dead. When you remove the nerve, the blood supply to the tooth is gone. Over time, because the tooth is dead and it is not receiving the nutrition from the blood supply, the tooth can become brittle. Teeth that have gone through root canals are more likely to fracture compared to healthy, natural teeth. One of the ways that dentists can help to avoid future problems with root canal teeth is to place a crown on the tooth. A crown is like putting a helmet on the tooth to hold it together and keep it from breaking. Sometimes we can even implant a post where the nerve used to be to help reinforce the tooth.

The Impact Of Teeth Grinding And Potential Treatments

Teeth grinding can be seriously detrimental to your mouth. Research indicates that clenching and grinding your teeth can make you susceptible to migraines and headaches. It can cause cracks and break down your teeth. It can also make your teeth more mobile, which means when you push on them they actually move. It can also increase your risk for periodontitis or gum disease.

This is the illustration that I use with patients: a fence post in the sand. If you were to use a sledgehammer to beat a fence post from side to side, eventually the sand would erode away from the bottom of the fence post, and the fence post would be loose. That is the same type of thing that happens to your teeth when you grind them. You are putting lateral forces on the teeth and the support structure. The teeth loosen up. Either the bones will give way or the tooth will give way. From a dental standpoint, it actually can be a pretty simple thing to deal with. Many times, it just requires the fabrication of a nighttime appliance that will prevent the patient from grinding teeth during any sleep cycle. There are several different types available, depending on the patient's needs.

I prefer the types that not only protect the teeth but also treat the neuromuscular part of the condition. The muscles are actually doing the clenching and grinding. The teeth do not make themselves come together. The muscles make your teeth come together and grind. Addressing muscle function, as well as protecting the teeth, is important when considering the type of appliance to use.

How Should You Pick Your Dentist?

I like this question, and it is one people often ask me. I begin my answer by telling them to find a dentist that they can trust—someone who makes them feel at home. This goes along with the premise of this book: your dentist should be someone with whom you would like to have a cup of coffee, someone with whom you would enjoy spending time. That is the key.

Even with the quality of dental school and licensing requirements, there can be some variation in the care that you receive, but the most important thing is for you to trust your dentist. If you trust your dentist, you know that if something does not go well, your dentist will tell you and address it. In the rare event that things may not go as planned, a trustworthy dentist will make sure that he or she addresses the problem or issue and takes care of it for the patient. You should never have to be concerned about whether or not you are receiving quality care if you trust the individual.

Find someone with a team that feels like family. You should feel the same way about the dentist's team as you do about the dentist. You should be comfortable with the assistant and the hygienist. You should be able to ask them questions and trust them as much as you do the dentist. A dental relationship is all about trust.

(This content should be used for informational purposes only. It does not create a doctor-patient relationship with any reader and should not be construed as medical advice. If you need medical advice, please contact a doctor in your community who can assess the specifics of your situation.)

5

A Compassionate, Gentle, and Honest Dental Practice

by Edita Outericka, D.M.D.

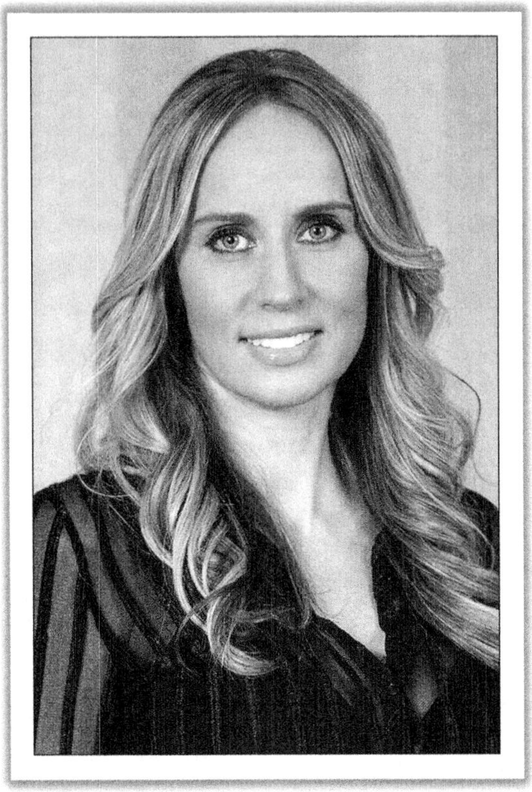

Edita Outericka, D.M.D.

Dynamic Dental, Inc.
Mansfield, Massachusetts
www.dynamicdentalinc.com

Dr. Edita Outericka, Dental Director at Dynamic Dental, strives for perfection and works tirelessly to educate patients on good overall dental health and proper dental hygiene. She has found cosmetic dentistry, including Invisalign (clear braces), most rewarding and has taken special interest in that area of her practice. Her enthusiasm for providing the highest quality dental care is matched only by the compassion she has for her patients. Dr. Edita graduated from Simmons College with a Bachelor's Degree and then entered the graduate program at Tufts University where she earned her Doctorate in Medical Dentistry. She is also certified to administer Botox and fillers. Dr. Edita is a member of both the American Dental Association and the Massachusetts Dental Society. She is also affiliated with the Southeastern Dental Society, South Shore District Dental Society and the New England Dental Society. When Dr. Edita is not working or spending time at dental seminars, she is an avid athlete who competes in triathlons and half marathons. She also supports charitable athletic events by raising money and participating in them. Dr. Edita currently resides in Easton with her husband.

A Compassionate, Gentle, and Honest Dental Practice

A Little Bit About Me

The greatest influence of my growing-up years was the journey that I experienced when my immediate family escaped from Europe to come to America. It definitely made me the person that I am today. In 1983, at ten years old, I came to the United States when my parents emigrated from the Czech Republic to Boston, Massachusetts. Of course, they wanted us to escape Communism, but they were mainly motivated by the opportunities that we could enjoy in the United States. When we arrived in the United States, we brought with us a total of $100. I respect my parents for sacrificing so much for their children. Both of my parents found jobs and worked hard so that after just one year, they could afford a home in Randolph, Massachusetts, as well as educations for my brother and me. As a family, we worked tirelessly to learn English and become Citizens—which we all did very quickly.

Academically, we were actually behind. While the schools in the Czech Republic were very good, English was a second language for us, so our education in the States began in classes for children who speak another language in their home. It was challenging, but it is a challenge I will never regret. In just a few years, with the help and devotion of my family, I was enrolled in advanced placement courses. Upon graduating high school, I enrolled at Simmons College in Boston. I received a scholarship to help pay for schooling and my parents contributed the rest of the money I needed for tuition and living expenses. I majored in and earned a Bachelor's Degree in Economics and Business. Once accepted, I looked forward to entering Tufts Dental School. It was really exciting to be accepted to the school of my choice. I really did not want to go anywhere else. It was definitely a challenging time with a lot of work, commit-ment, and cost; but it was all worth it! I have enjoyed this field so much.

By the time I turned 13 years old, I knew I wanted to become a dentist. I wanted to help people and I was fascinated by teeth and working with my mind and meticulously using my hands. My first job was as an assistant in an orthodontist's office. I then had numerous other jobs as a dental assistant, which put me slightly ahead of my classmates in dental school. Now, I am living my own version of the American dream right here in a practice that was built on the fundamentals I live by.

My Philosophy Of Dentistry

I believe in providing the highest quality health care to my patients. This is accomplished by using leading-edge, modern high-tech equipment and concentrating on patient satisfaction. In the office, we treat people the way any person would want to be treated—with compassion, gentleness, and kindness. You have to do the right thing. You must be honest. At the end of the day, you have to be able to put your head down on the pillow and just feel good about what you did. That is the philosophy that I live by in my practice.

I am also a fan of continuing education and being open to learning new procedures that may provide a higher level of care or make for a more comfortable patient experience. We need to be willing to try out new ideas along with the corresponding new technology in order to provide the very best possible care for our patients. That is the mindset I have instilled in my practice and it is the way we train our team. Everyone must be committed to this philosophy without compromise.

The Importance Of Preventive Dentistry

I am a huge advocate of preventive dental care for children. Parents are being urged by their primary care physicians to take their children in for dental visits. This should be done early and often to establish good health habits and catch problems ahead of time. Previously, dentists saw children for the first time at around four or five years old. Now, we want children coming into the office for a checkup at age one. By starting early, we can help them become acclimated to the office and at ease sitting in the chair—all this while exposing them to dental routines. Children will become comfortable with the dental visit, and as they grow, they will come as often as they should.

People tend to forget the importance of the oral cavity's connection to the rest of the body. The presence of decay, bacteria, plaque, tartar, an abscess, and infection can send bacteria throughout your entire body. The health of your mouth can affect your heart, your arteries/veins, the health of an unborn child—everything. One of the biggest reasons for practicing preventive care from a young age is to avoid those ill effects of oral decay.

Early Diagnosis Helps In Successful Treatment Plans

Often, the signs of the body's systemic problems show up first in the mouth. Oral cancer comes to mind immediately. If a dentist can catch a mouth condition at an early stage, before other symptoms develop, it can be prevented from growing into a very traumatic issue, potentially throughout the body. Oral cancer screening is a very important reason to visit your dentist!

People who have trouble with their TMJ, such as jaw pain that causes headaches and migraines, often turn to a reliance on pills and medication instead of dealing with the problem. Eventually, that becomes a vicious cycle. Getting biopsies on oral lesions to screenings for oral cancer are not things people can treat on their own. If a patient visits the dentist once every five years because of an existing problem or embedded pain, it might already be too late. Come regularly, get thorough evaluations, and try to catch problems at an early stage when something can be done about it.

Collaboration With Other Doctors

In my area of practice, health care providers regularly meet to discuss our concerns as well as the new trends and treatments that we see. More eyes on the problem is best, especially when a doctor is trained in a specific field of expertise. We are able to get a much more complete picture by discussing complex cases with specialists and other doctors. As professionals, we compare notes and refer back and forth as necessary. This is better for our patients. If I think that the patient's primary doctor should look at something, I will send the patient without hesitation. Most primary care physicians also ask these questions as a matter of course: "When was the last time that you had a dental check-up? When did you last see your dentist for any treatment?" This is part of maintaining good health.

If anything in the patient's answers seem problematic to the primary care physician, they will say, "Please make an appointment to see a dentist now. Here is your referral, I will follow up with you if you do not." Some doctors will send us a letter or email saying, "Hey, I referred a patient that I am concerned about; he has not seen a dentist for a while. Could you please follow up?" We are working together to address the problem and making it easier for patients to come in and be seen. That is the way health care should work.

Now, because so much information is available to doctors and patients alike, I think that people are taking a more proactive approach to healthcare. Patients are bombarded with information about the importance of being attuned to their health. Doctors and dentists blog about concerns and issues; people get to see these topics online and on TV. Media coverage has definitely increased the flow of people actually coming into the office and being more concerned about their health.

Building A Healthcare Team That Works

The philosophy of our office is focused on meeting the needs of the patients in the best way that we can. We stay open late or on weekends to make it easier for busy people to get convenient appointments. We attempt to match the doctor's personality to the team members and the patients. Since I could not possibly see patients from 8 A.M. to 8 P.M. by myself, our first goal was to find exceptional dentists whom we could train and work with—those who work in the way that we want our practice to operate. We brought in the dentist and the team that came along with him or her, including the assistants and hygienists. Our entire team was hired based on the principle of providing high quality treatment and accommodating our patients.

Since we want our patients to be comfortable with us, we screen the patients in order to place them with a dentist whose style would suit the patient. If a patient can only come in at seven o'clock at night, we are able to give him that seven o'clock appointment with a doctor who will connect with him and meet his special needs.

My role is to facilitate and foster this association so that the arrangement continues to work smoothly. While I am also able to do actual dentistry and see my own patients on certain days, I love meeting and training people, especially in the clinical aspect. I actually enjoy the business side of dentistry, which is not usual for most dentists, though I will need to find the right person to take over the directorial side of the practice as we grow. Being up front with the staff and training them in our way of doing things can make this whole connection flow more easily. It is our goal to ensure a pleasant patient experience with every team member, so we spend a lot of time and attention on training.

Our philosophy is paying off. After starting this business in 2009, we outgrew our place within one year. It was just crazy—in a good way—and we are still growing. As you grow from five patients to 100 times that number of patients, it is necessary to make some changes and accommodate the growth, while still paying attention to every patient and making each one number one. No one can do it alone; you must have a committed team. We have been able to do just that. I am not saying we never stumble. Sometimes it is a rollercoaster, but we learn from our shortcomings. We improve and pursue our goals again.

We will be expanding into a bigger space this year, which will accommodate everyone. The next challenge involves our expansion: putting systems into place to accommodate the upcoming changes. You always have to go with the growth and adapt to the changes. Keeping up with the constant flow makes it very easy for the patient.

KEEPING RADIATION AT A MINIMUM

Many patients ask why we take X-rays. They say, "I do not want to be exposed to radiation." One of the first things that we do is to explain how X-rays have changed over to digital X-rays; the exposure is faster, more focused, and minimal. Then, we try to agree with the patient on how the X-ray issue will be handled. "We will take X-rays once a year for diagnosis. We are going to take bitewings this time and then full sets of X-rays next time."

I take X-rays when I feel that it is beneficial for proper diagnosis, on an individual patient-by-patient basis. If the patient has a history of rampant decay, or does not take care of oral hygiene and I cannot see the problem simply by looking into his or her mouth, then I will take an X-ray. That could mean every two weeks, every three months, or once every six months. The frequency depends upon the individual. As a basic rule, I would say that X-rays are needed, on average, once per year. That basic rule is not set in stone. You simply cannot expect every patient to follow the same treatment path. Every patient should be treated individually based upon his dental history and specific need.

Cosmetic Considerations

I get cosmetic dental questions all the time. Questions include topics such as, "How do I make my teeth look better if I do not want to wear braces?" Many older patients who have previously had braces or other metal appliances will object to a second installation, saying, "I have to work with people face-to-face and I do not want to wear anything metal on my teeth." Again, before offering treatment options, the dentist must get to know the patient, his expectations, his circumstances, and his budget.

There are numerous ways to improve a person's smile. It is possible for a dentist to re-shape and polish a patient's teeth to make them look better, which is the least costly way. It is great if you know that your patient will be satisfied with just that procedure. However, if your patient wants something better and has the time and money, other options include veneers, crowns, Invisalign® (clear, nearly invisible retainer braces in the mouth), or special bonding. In my opinion, patients just need personalized guidance in terms of the best treatment for them, depending on what they are willing to put into the process of treatment.

A great smile can be a big factor when it comes to family, your appearance in photographs, your confidence, and your relationships in business and social situations. Of course, if the patient wants his smile corrected, as a dentist, you have to listen to what he is saying and accommodate him in the best way that you can without jeopardizing his health or providing unnecessary treatment. The end goal is to make the smile right so that both the doctor and the patient are happy with the results.

To Seal Or Not To Seal

We tell parents of those children who are not candidates for sealants, "No, there is really no need for sealants." Some kids definitely do a great job with hygiene; they do not need to have sealants on their teeth. At our office, many parents also ask about the safety of putting sealants on their children's teeth—what it involves, how it works. Sometimes, they are concerned about putting chemicals on their children's teeth. Of course, we take the time to answer all of their questions. For instance, we let parents know that there are different kinds of sealants; some include fluoride release and some do not. If you are one of those parents who do not like having fluoride in your child's mouth, you can choose a sealant without the fluoride.

Also, if sealants are not placed properly, they can actually do more damage than good. If a child has deep grooves in his teeth, it is very difficult to clean those grooves properly, we might consider sealants. If there are stains in the grooves, and the child is struggling to keep his teeth healthy, we may recommend placing sealants but only if we can first remove some of that staining and bacteria. After being sure the surface is clean and clear, we would seal those grooves properly, making it easier for the child to prevent decay in the future. If the grooves are minimal, and the child is cleaning his teeth properly, then sealants are not always recommended because the child is already doing the sealant's job.

If the parents and their dentist decide to use sealants, it is important that the area is properly cleaned. That involves the dentist using a small pin-point drill to clean out any staining and decay-causing bacteria that might be in the groove. The sealant must also be applied properly and completely, with no access for bacteria to grow underneath. Once bacteria gets embedded underneath, it is hard to diagnose. It could actually blow up into a huge decay problem, even leading to a root canal. Sealants should be carefully rechecked at every appointment when patients come in for their regular visits. If there is any chipping, voids, or staining, sealant should be replaced as soon as possible.

Fillings – Correcting The Past And Improving The Future

In the past, all dentists used silver fillings. As you probably know, they last a very long time. These silver fillings are still working on patients who had them placed 20 to 25 years ago. We do not have to go in and replace the silver fillings on every person who comes in the door.

Tooth-colored fillings have come a long way, but every material has its pros and cons. Tooth-colored fillings are becoming more popular because many patients do not want to see silver when they open their mouths. They want white to match their teeth, so that "no one will know I had a cavity." The demand for white fillings now outweighs the demand for silver fillings.

Some patients will make cost-based decisions—silver fillings are less expensive. In our office, we make the decision based on what is right for your tooth. The silver filling is packed into the tooth with a lot of force, and it is based on retention of the preparation for the silver filling. A lot of patching goes into the walls of the tooth to make sure that the filling will adhere, and then the material hardens. The filling itself is made up of different types of metals so when it hardens, it is pretty strong.

The initial issue with the silver filling is that it contracts and expands. That makes the tooth slightly fluctuate in and out, causing little cracks in the teeth. Over the lifetime of the filling, the patient will develop cracks in his teeth that get bigger and bigger. Dentists are now seeing lots of cracked teeth from old silver fillings because as you are chewing with your teeth, the cracks expand. As those cracks get bigger, a patient can eventually crack his whole tooth and then the repair involves a different treatment.

Tooth-colored fillings can still have some leakage at the meeting point of the chewing forces. The white filling can wear off, so the anatomical shape of the tooth is lost because of the grinding-down of the filling over time. By contrast, the silver filling keeps that nice anatomy because of the strength of the material. Tooth-colored filling bonding, if it is done well and isolated properly without exposure to moisture, can also last a very long time. These days, it is bonded to the tooth so it avoids that tooth-cracking process.

The bottom line comes down to cracking. While silver fillings are strong, they have the negative effect of cracking your whole tooth over time. White fillings, on the other hand, are bonded to your tooth. This means they must be placed precisely and bonded perfectly. These fillings must look good alongside the natural tooth-color—the shade you select which matches the tooth. Then the filling looks beautiful.

Our office mostly places tooth-colored bonded fillings because of our patients' preferences. If there were a procedure in which tooth-colored fillings might not be appropriate, then we would consider an alternative; we do not just place something because a patient wants it. Silver fillings will eventually become unavailable, partially because of the metal inside, since mercury is used as part of the amalgam. People are more concerned about mercury these days than they were in the past. We are required to separate out any amalgam we extract when we remove silver fillings. This is done to keep the mercury out of the environment and allow it to be disposed of properly.

Options For Teeth Whitening

When it comes to teeth whitening, some patients arrive and say, "I know what I want. This is what I want to do." Our office reviews the options in detail with them: the whitening systems, the requirements for each system, the prices, etc. Most of the time, we know the patient's dental history, sensitivities, the kinds of staining on the teeth, and existing dental work. For instance, if he or she has heavy staining or fillings, we let him know that it might be necessary to replace the fillings to match the whitening process of his actual teeth. We know each patient well enough to anticipate his or her expectations.

All of these things affect their decisions regarding whitening. We provide preparation materials ahead of time, such as special pre-bleaching toothpaste, so we can then recommend a "bleaching system" and they will be happy with the results. We work toward the best treatment for that patient. For example, it could be the fast in-office Zoom!® system, which only requires the patient to sit in the chair for about an hour.

A "whitening system" is a longer process than any in-office bleaching system, and it takes place over a period of time. Most patients do not have the time to do that. They want it done quickly. As a dentist, you have to explain the consequences to them.

Sometimes, in order to get whiter teeth, dentists have to take more aggressive steps to expose the patient to effective bleaching. Those steps cause a little more sensitivity than a whitening system would. Additionally, an in-office treatment is more expensive compared to the other options. Some patients could combine an in-office treatment with take-home bleaching trays to get the best results. For others who have the patience to do their own bleaching, we can provide trays so that they can do it at home over a two-week period of time. Younger patients with more sensitive teeth might receive something simpler, like over-the-counter Crest® strips.

The Options For Replacing Missing Teeth

In the past patients would say, "I went to the dentist and they just pulled my tooth; now, I have a space here." It is true that is was common for dentists extract a tooth rather than trying to save it.

People need their teeth to chew, smile, retain the bones of the jaw and provide shape and structure to their face. Today, people are more conscious of their teeth. They want missing teeth to be replaced and they want the new tooth to perfectly match their existing natural teeth. The options are based on the patient's finances and the ongoing mouth situation in terms of bone loss, the contouring of the gingiva, and a number of other factors. Once those factors have been evaluated, a decision can be made to place an implant, a bridge, partials, or dentures. There are many attractive options with amazing success rates. The dentist should explain to the patient all of the pros and cons of each one beyond just the cost.

Implants are the most expensive of those options. Before a dentist can place an individual prosthetic tooth, he must first see if the patient even qualifies for the procedure. For instance, the patient must have the enough bone available in their mouth for this procedure. The patient's dental history is also really important, including any history of smoking or current nicotine usage. If the patient qualifies for an implant, an implant screw (which will integrate into the bone over time) is placed into the jawbone. That screw is left in place for eight to twelve weeks; if the screw successfully stays in, the dentist can actually place a tooth on that implant. It functions like a natural tooth. You can chew on it, bite with it, and treat it like your own tooth. It will not come off. It is there permanently. In my opinion, implants are the best option for a qualified patient to replace missing teeth.

Bridges would probably be the second most costly item after the implants. The patient must have adjacent and healthy teeth in order to hold a bridge. If one tooth is not healthy or anything happens to one part of that bridge, that whole bridge will fail. A bridge is a permanent appliance that rests on multiple healthy teeth. It is essential to also look at the patient's dental history and determine his dental health before qualifying him for the procedure.

The least expensive way to replace missing teeth is with a partial or denture. These are removable appliances. Patients must take them out, clean them, and take care of them. They are made of acrylic-porcelain, so they can crack. The appliances may need to be replaced or realigned to remain comfortable and properly positioned.

Processes are now available to place implants underneath the denture and lock the dentures in place so that they do not move at all. This is used instead of the more common method of using suction to hold them in place. This approach becomes a little more costly. Ultimately, it depends on the patient's expectations, financial situation, and options for a proper fit, given the history of the mouth. Once again, spending time with the patient to decide on the best treatment is the best way to proceed with solving any problem. A missing tooth is no longer something that you just have to live with.

Gum Disease Has Serious Health Consequences

Periodontal disease is another daily problem for dentists. In our practice, when our patients arrive for their first visit, they have a comprehensive exam with the doctor. The patients also see the hygienist. The hygienist does a thorough cleaning. Every patient has probing and x-rays done if they are due and necessary.

The doctor sees the patient for a thorough evaluation which includes oral cancer screening, looking at existing restorations, evaluating the probing depths and x-rays, and establishing treatment plans for the future. The patient meets the doctor(s) during the initial appointment, and there is time for questions.

During the comprehensive exam combined and using the information from the hygienist, we determine the level of gum disease for every patient. Obviously, if we say, "everything is great," patients do not have to come back until their next appointment in six months. If gum disease is present, we address it right away. There are several stages of the gum disease, gingivitis being the mildest form and ranging to the most serious condition—Type 4 Periodontitis.

At that first exam, we discover where patients stand as far as gum health and determine the necessary treatment. We also look at the patient's history. If they have had regular cleanings, but they still show Type 1 Gingivitis, that usually requires a good cleaning and a re-evaluation in three to four months. Sometimes, if that Type 1 Gingivitis is not addressed by the patient at home, then gingivitis leads to the next stage—Type 2 Periodontitis.

This progression means that regular brushing and flossing at home is not getting rid of the bacteria. It is too deeply embedded for the toothbrush to get in there and clean it out. Therefore, patients need our help to get into the deeper areas and clean out the bacteria. Depending upon the pocketing—how deeply our probe extends into the pocket—some patients might need three to five visits to handle the problem. We can determine where we will do more aggressive treatment than a regular cleaning. With the two- or three-millimeter pockets, we just review oral hygiene practices and go into some improvements. When a patient has four- to six-millimeter pockets, they will actually need to return to the office for a treatment under local anesthesia. Once they get numb (because they would feel discomfort), we go into the pocket and clean out the bacteria that the patient or the regular cleaning is not able to reach.

As soon as that bacteria is cleaned out, patients must maintain the health of that pocket for another three months; that means visiting their dentist every three months to keep the pocket clean. Otherwise, bacteria will burrow deeper and deeper by eating away at the bone that holds the teeth together. If that deterioration continues, teeth become mobile or loose. That is how we lose teeth. We cannot make your bone grow back, but we can stabilize the deterioration so that it does not get worse. The level of bone health or deterioration is how we determine the treatment. The next step is the deep cleaning, meaning scaling and root planing, in order to clean all the way to the roots. This procedure requires you to be numb because the cleaning is a much more aggressive form of treatment. Once the bacteria is removed, we can maintain the pockets every three months for you and the condition should not get worse.

If the patient does not attend regular visits every three months (this is a big problem), prolongs the time between visits, or does not come in at all, the condition will regress. Soon you are starting all over again with the same problems, or worse. If the condition gets worse, then we might have to refer you to a specialist (periodontist) who could treat by doing a surgical procedure to move your gums out of the way in order to clean out all of the bacteria. Afterward, you would be on protocol maintenance, maybe alternating between a periodontist and your hygienist. It just depends on each individual's situation. Most multi-specialty practices have a periodontist in the same practice.

As dentists, we try to catch these situations ahead of time to prevent the problems from escalating. If the same bacteria go unattended, bacteria involved in the plaque and tartar at the gum line, and do not get cleaned off by regular cleanings, then they will travel through your entire body. Also, sometimes tartar buildup is so hardened on the teeth that it resists the hygienists' probe (the measurement device), and the measurement of the problem is not diagnosed early enough. Occasionally, it is necessary to remove the tartar and bacteria ahead of time just to access, measure, and diagnose the mouth issues correctly.

The same bacteria found in your mouth can also be found in your arteries and affects your heart; it can cause damage throughout your whole body, not just your mouth. That is why dentists are so very adamant about diagnosing periodontal disease properly, catching it at the early stages, and maintaining dental health. It is a huge part of what a dentist does because bacteria buildup can affect the patient's overall health.

TEETH GRINDING IS A COMMON PROBLEM

A great number of patients come into the office and complain about symptoms of Bruxism, or teeth grinding. They might say, "My jaw is sore and hurting me," or, "I have chronic headaches," or, "I have pain in the joint of my jaw," or, "My teeth are wearing down. Why is that?"

There are a number of reasons people grind, but it is generally stress-related, and grinding almost always happens while the person is asleep. There is a genetic component, and the alignment of your teeth and mandibular joint also comes into play. You may have some clenching issues during the day when you are stressed at work or while driving; you might be clenching your teeth without even realizing it. Most of it, though, is done during sleep; the patient is oblivious until they come in with a complaint.

We start by examining the teeth for signs of grinding. Then we look at the different options for treatment. Depending upon the level of pain, as far as headaches and joint pain, there can be several levels of treatment.

First, we start patients with a special guard. Different types of guards address different situations. The type of guard used depends on the patient's history of crowns or other dental work in his or her mouth, his compliance level, the way he will wear it, and possible gag areas. That is when we decide on the appliance that will be best, from a guard that covers just the top teeth or the bottom teeth, to a full guard that covers all of the teeth. The guard can be soft or hard. We can also create smaller appliances if the patient tends to gag. Each appliance is custom-made to fit that patient's teeth. Typically, the appliance is worn at night. Usually, the price range is from $300 to $800.

The goal of the appliance is to align the teeth properly, so that eventually you will not grind anymore. There are ways to mask the grinding and prevent the teeth from wearing down, but the real goal should be to find an appliance that helps you to properly align your jaw and teeth. Other steps can be taken if that does not solve the problem, such as referring a patient to a TMJ specialist for splints or a surgery, but you always want to start with the appliance, which usually solves the problem. Should the appliance work, the patient will feel much better because his teeth are not wearing down and the pain and migraines/headaches go away. If the grinding issues are solved or prevented before the teeth crack and the restorations fail, this can save a patient thousands of dollars and a lot of multi-procedure trauma.

Protecting Your Teeth Is Important

When your children participate in sports, having the right mouth guard is important for them. The "right" sports guard is chosen to work with the children's history. For example, it is customized so that they can wear it if they have braces. Of course, there are also considerations over which sports they play, their history of gagging or not gagging, and several other factors. Sports guards are not a one-size-fits-all situation. We custom-make the right appliance for that patient to use during the sports they participate in and based on a number of other determining factors.

The sports guard works in a similar manner to that of a night guard. I think that a lot of parents need to be more educated about their kids' sports and coaches' checklists. Some are required to wear sports guards at times but not always. I am working with some of the local sports teams now to determine the best plan for preventing injury. In the professional sports world, guards are mandatory. That might be something to consider for younger players, too.

Sedation Dentistry Can Help Overcome Dental Fears

Apart from nitrous oxide and Valium, we do not yet provide sedation dentistry in our office. We try not to because we hope to win that patient over by working with them to decrease their fear and anxiety. Dentistry should not hurt. I do not believe that patients should ever be uncomfortable in the chair. I try to show patients slowly, step by step, that they can be comfortable when they walk in—no matter what that takes; 99.9% of the time, we succeed and the patients learn to trust that we will not hurt them.

Occasionally, a dentist might need some of these sedation aids in the beginning of the relationship with the patient, especially if the patient has had a previous bad experience. It is difficult to work on a patients who are tense and fearful because they will not open their mouth. If the dentist cannot access their oral cavity, how can he or she provide the proper treatment? The biggest benefit of sedation dentistry, including nitrous oxide and Valium, is that dentists can provide the necessary care without the difficulty of accessing the oral cavity properly.

In the most common type of sedation dentistry, patients do not remember anything after the treatment, even if they moved around or made noises during the procedure. A "bite block" is inserted to keep the mouth open, so the assistant and dentist can get into the oral cavity and preventing the patient from closing the mouth. Most offices have the necessary equipment and staff to offer more options, including an anesthesiologist with special training or a visiting sedation dentist.

Choosing The Dentist That Is Right For You

Obviously, the best way to choose a dentist is a recommendation from a friend, a family member, or somebody who has had a good experience. Many patients rely on the Internet, searching through Google. I would also urge any patient to find the answers to a few questions. Is the office modern, with high-tech equipment? Do the dentists and support staff keep up with current procedures? Call and ask the office these questions or at least search for public reviews. Are the reviews positive, and what do they say? Is the facility clean? All of this information can make you feel better about choosing a dentist.

Also, look for an office that is open during convenient hours. Patients have jobs and they need to work. Your health care team should accommodate your schedule to some extent. It is not productive if the patient wants to take good care of her teeth, but there is no open office time for her to come in. Also, make sure that the office accepts your dental insurance. Too often, patients call an office and hear, "No, we do not take insurance anymore." These patients finally have the benefits of dental insurance through their job, but they are not able to use it. That is very frustrating.

Another big consideration is to find an office that provides multiple services. It is so nice when you are able to connect with a team, you like them, and you can get everything that you need without being sent elsewhere. Many patients do not want to be sent out or referred out to another place. They want their whole team in one spot. It helps patients—particularly the ones who fear dental visits—to feel more secure. Having these multi-specialty practices under one roof is an excellent benefit for patients. This can be hugely important for families who are able to bring their child to the same dental office that they themselves visit. If you meet an individual dentist whose philosophy or ideas do not mesh with yours, sometimes it is necessary to say, "I am sorry, this probably is not going to work for either of us." Both parties need to feel that connection.

When you get to the bottom line, you need to understand the importance of your oral health in relation to your overall health. You need to protect your oral health. The same is true for your children. Find a dentist who will help you reach this goal. Be sure that treatment is presented in a way that keeps you and your children coming back for regular visits. Regular visits, keeping up with oral hygiene at home and treating issues early are the keys to great oral health.

(This content should be used for informational purposes only. It does not create a doctor-patient relationship with any reader and should not be construed as medical advice. If you need medical advice, please contact a doctor in your community who can assess the specifics of your situation.)

6

Our Golden Rule: Comprehensive Care Without Cutting Corners

by Patricia E. Takacs, D.M.D.

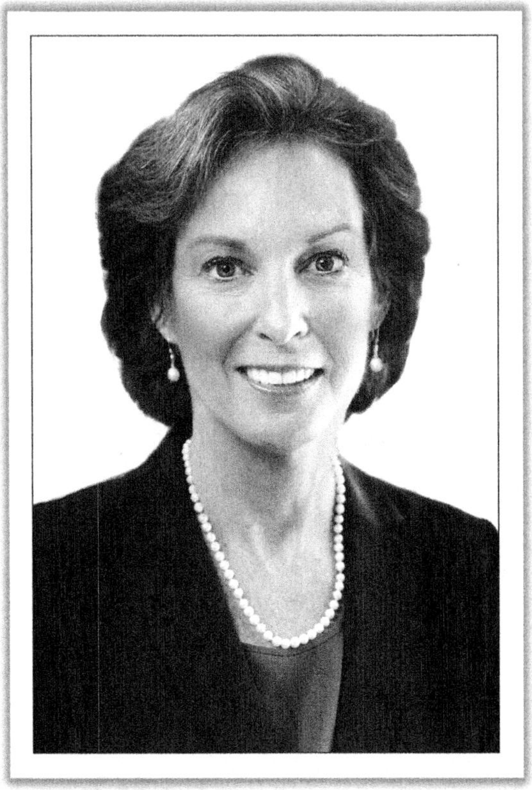

Patricia E. Takacs, D.M.D.

Beaumont Family Dentistry
Lexington, Kentucky
www.beaumontfamilydentistry.com

Dr. Patricia Takacs opened her first practice over 30 years ago with the purpose to reach out to everyone and improve their dental health in a comfortable, modern environment. Dr. Takacs is a strong advocate of patient education and enjoys getting to know each of her patients.

She is dedicated to staying current with cutting-edge procedures and technology. She has completed advanced training in implant dentistry, neuromuscular analysis, orthodontics, cosmetic dentistry, full mouth reconstruction and sleep apnea medicine. She is trained and certified in oral conscious sedation. As an Elite Preferred Invisalign Provider, Dr. Takacs has the highest status as an Invisalign provider and is in the top 1% of all providers in North America. She is also a Lumineers-certified doctor.

After attending West Virginia University, Dr. Takacs graduated with honors from the University of Kentucky, College of Dentistry in 1983. In addition to running her practice, she has taught at the University of Kentucky, College of Dentistry and coached dentists through a dental management company.

A Member of Academy of GP Orthodontics, Academy of Laser Dentistry, Academy of Computerized Dentistry, Bluegrass Dental Society, Kentucky Dental Association, American Dental Association and Dental Organization of Conscious Sedation.

Dr. Trish Takacs and her husband have been married 33 years and have a son and daughter. Her son is a 2012 graduate of UK College of Dentistry and is an associate at Beaumont Family Dentistry and her daughter will be graduating from the Dental College in 2015. Her outside interests include golf and reading and hanging out with the family dogs.

OUR GOLDEN RULE: COMPREHENSIVE CARE WITHOUT CUTTING CORNERS

DENTISTRY HAS ALWAYS BEEN A PART OF MY LIFE

My childhood was very, very stable; my parents were married for more than 49 years before my dad's death in 2003. My mom stayed at home, so we always had somebody there when we got home from school. I have two older brothers, and I was kind of a tomboy. They'd ask me to step in to bat on the baseball team or join in on a pickup game of basketball or football. I played any sort of sport, from golf to softball. A big difference between these days and my growing-up years is that we could ride our bikes anywhere without worrying; we may not see those days again.

Academics and sports were an important part of my growing up years. My brothers and I all played high school sports and we all graduated either as first or second in our respective classes. My parents definitely pushed education; the agreement with my father was that he would pay for us to go to college, but beyond that, we were responsible to pay for any continuing education. My oldest brother graduated with a mechanical engineering degree from Purdue University and lives in Richmond, Virginia. My middle brother is an attorney in Nashville, Tennessee, having gone to Notre Dame and Vanderbilt Law School. I attended West Virginia University and graduated with Honors from the University of Kentucky College of Dentistry in 1983.

Dentistry has been an important part of my life since I was a child. My mother's dad was a dentist in Munster, Indiana, which is just outside of Chicago. He was a major influence on my decision to become a dentist. Before moving from Indiana, I would spend hours at my grandfather's office getting into his "treasure chest" and riding the pump up chairs or watching him wax up dentures. He loved what he did and I loved going to his office. Now, since both of my children (my son and my daughter) have decided to go into dentistry, we essentially have a family practice. Even my mother works in the office keeping everybody comfortable—she brings the patients coffee and cookies. (Yes, cookies. I'll explain later.)

When I started third grade, we moved to Vienna, West Virginia. I spent most of my learning years in West Virginia. I graduated from high school in 1976 and began my first year at WVU. After completing my first year with the intention of going to dental school, my mother asked if I, as a female, really wanted to become a dentist. "Why don't you become a physical therapist? You can set your own hours." After changing my major to physical therapy, in my second year, I changed back to biology—physical therapy just wasn't a good fit. After my junior year at WVU, I interviewed at University of Kentucky and got accepted to the University of Kentucky College of Dentistry in Lexington, Kentucky.

I met my husband-to-be in Lexington—it's kind of a weird story but fun, too. During my first year in dental school, I was rooming with my across-the-street neighbor from West Virginia. She was a nurse at the hospital which also housed the dental school. She had gone to college in Niagara Falls, New York. My husband is from Buffalo, and was at Niagara at the same time. He actually was dating my friend from West Virginia's old roommate. He got a job at the Hyatt Regency in Dallas and got transferred to the Lexington Hyatt Regency during my first year at dental school. He called up my roommate and she invited him to our apartment.

We both knew that we were going to get married as soon as we met. We have been married since 1981.

I graduated from dental school in 1983 and my husband decided to go to law school in 1984. Our son was born in 1985, during my husband's first year of law school and five months after I opened my own dental practice. Our daughter was born in 1988 when we were both working. I won't say that it has all been clear sailing. In my early years, I remember that sensation of ice-cold fear, thinking that maybe I was going to lose everything. Starting a business and building a practice is very expensive, and it doesn't happen overnight. Most importantly, I knew that if my practice was successful, my kids wouldn't have to wade through the same hard times as I did.

I wasn't originally from Kentucky—I was a newly-minted dentist who had to establish my practice from the ground up. Now, we have three separate successful offices in the Lexington area that are all doing well. My son graduated from UKCD in 2012 and joined my practice. My daughter graduated from UK College of Dentistry in 2015. Our "family practice" is set. We have an excellent set of values, a solid mission, and a vision for the future. I know that there are many more opportunities as far as building referral networks to bring in patients with both internal and external marketing. I work with a great team of dentists, hygienists, assistants, and front office personnel so this dream is very attainable—and very exciting. We have a three-year plan; now we just have to work it.

Not Just Tooth Doctors—Physicians Of The Mouth

I've always felt that everybody deserves to have access to quality dental care that is also affordable. At Beaumont Family Dentistry, we take care of our patients as we would expect to be taken care of as patients; the Golden Rule applies in each of our offices. We provide optimal care without cutting corners. If our patients don't have the money for a procedure, or if they're on a restrictive insurance plan, we still provide the same quality of care. We help each of our patients find the means to afford dental care, often using third party financing with very low to zero interest rates. We even have created our own in-office insurance plan for our patients who have no coverage. Comprehensive dental care is very important. It shouldn't be sacrificed due to cost.

Educating our patients is one of our biggest responsibilities. People need to understand the connection between the health of your mouth and the health of your body. If you have gum disease, for example, the bacteria in your mouth are spreading infection throughout your entire body. If your teeth are not properly aligned or you are grinding your teeth while you sleep, it can eventually affect your ability to properly chew and digest your food. Clenching, grinding or bruxing while you sleep puts extreme pressure on your teeth and also on your jaw. This can lead to discomfort, pain, headaches, and even tooth fracture or loss. These problems all have causes that can be diagnosed and treated—so there is really no need to suffer. However, you have to do the first part—come into our office (where you will be rewarded with cookies).

I truly believe that dentistry should be recognized as a specialty of medicine. It is amazing to realize the number of links and interactions between what we do and what medical doctors (MDs) do. There are many diseases and conditions that occur orally which can cause medical problems elsewhere in the body. There are also many telltale symptoms and signs to be found orally that are indicative of existing medical problems elsewhere.

Dentists are often the first to spot them and therefore refer to the patient's medical doctor. Dentists and MDs can work together and more interactively in the mutual care of our patients.

An oral cancer screening is one of the most important exams that we do for our patients. This exam should be performed by every dentist as well as hygienists. If oral cancer is not diagnosed early, the morbidity and mortality rates are high. We have incorporated the use of a VELscope® as part of the oral cancer screening exam. First, there is the clinical part, in which we visually look at the structures in the mouth, palpating the neck and the lymph nodes. Then we use the VELscope® to check oral tissues to make sure that nothing looks suspicious with that different kind of lighting. Without the VELscope®, it is difficult to identify much of a visual difference in the tissues. So, we do that for every patient—it's very important. We have never discovered any major cancers, but we've seen suspicious areas and have referred patients for biopsies.

Medical Doctors and dentists are beginning to work together to ensure the overall health of the individual patient. This is particularly evident with dentist referrals to ENTs, Pediatrics, and cardiologists. In turn, we have seen many referrals to our practice for sleep disorder breathing and tongue tied infant treatment.

At Beaumont Family Dentistry, our mission is to provide, with empathy, the best in high-quality dental care to our patients. We treat each other and every patient as an individual. Therefore, we diagnose for any problems and create a treatment plan specifically for that individual in order to achieve our goals and functions. It's our role to treat every patient and each other with respect just as we expect to be treated. We strive to provide care and compassion for each patient from the initial phone contact to the completion of the required comprehensive dental treatment. Our vision is to create a workplace that is both fun and exciting, bringing each of us a sense of personal fulfillment, joy, and pride in our work. We work to develop a positive, nurturing, and safe environment so that our workday is comfortable and energized. We are committed to mutual respect, clear communication, and teamwork with each other.

For our patients, our goal is to provide a patient experience that exceeds their expectations in every area of contact. In the end, when our patients go out the door with optimal oral health, they're likely to refer their friends and family to our practice. Every day, we must live the vision of our practice in order to keep it alive and well.

Our commitment to continuing education is one way of keeping alive our vision and our goals. I feel that everybody who works at Beaumont Family Dentistry must be educated yearly. I make it a point that everybody gets continuing education to learn the trends and see what's up-and-coming. You can't stay ahead if half of your team stays behind. So, my assistants go with me when I go to my trainings; when I come back, I don't have to re-teach them. That's how I've always felt. I've also trained my team of dentists to take their staff with them to continuing education. I know that this is critically important and I cannot stress it enough.

Dental Problems And Sleep Apnea

Every staff member within the practice must have their fingers on the pulse of dentistry and the way it relates to the whole body. For example, due to continuing education, I have discovered that there is a key link between sleep apnea and oral health. I have attended various workshops focused on discovering craniofacial pain and its relationship with sleep apnea. It's a fascinating area that many physicians are not as aware of. And unfortunately, there's more to helping treat patients with sleep apnea than just being able to say, "Yes, I'm going to put you in an appliance." Education with the specialists in sleep medicine is paramount to being able, as dentists, to successfully treat our patients.

I have done much training in the realm of sleep apnea, sleep medicine, and sleep dentistry. I am a member of the American Academy of Dental Sleep Medicine, the American Academy of Sleep Medicine, and I also belong to the American Academy of Craniofacial Pain. I have completed a mini-residency at Tufts University in Sleep Medicine and Dentistry. We are becoming aware that sleep apnea causes a whole realm of medical problems that most people don't know anything about. Sleep apnea can lead to an increased risk of stroke, high blood pressure, heart attack, Type 2 diabetes, gastroesophageal reflux disease (GERD), fibromyalgia, atrial fibrillation (A-Fib), dementia, and ultimately, premature death. These medical issues occur because the person ceases to breathe for more than 10 seconds repeatedly during sleep. The number of times that this happens increases the risk of all of these factors that I've just mentioned.

To help our patients live longer, healthier lives, we teach the importance of healthy gums and teeth (to prevent heart disease, stroke, and increased blood pressure), and then assess potential underlying sleep problems. We also provide enhanced esthetics to improve self-esteem and appearance and virtually change someone's life. We improve the ability to function, eat, and speak. We are forever challenged by the myriad of medicines our patients take in order to control their medical problems. Many patients are completely unaware that they may have sleep apnea, but more importantly, why their dentist is recommending they be seen by their physician. Our role is to assess whether or not our patients might have an underlying sleep problem. The patient questionnaires cover important topics: how they sleep, whether they feel rested during the day, whether they snore, whether they gasp, whether others hear these things. Do they have headaches and jaw pain, or do they make noises at night? We look at their medical history and the types of medicines that they are taking. If they're taking two different blood pressure medicines or diabetic medicine, we are going to ask how they sleep. We provide an in-depth dental and medical history.

An oral exam will include evaluating wear on teeth, both the back teeth and the edges of the front teeth. Wear may indicate grinding and attempting to open their airway and bring their tongue forward as they move their lower jaw forward. I also look for evidence of GERD, which can show up like little pockets or potholes on the cusps of your molars. Shiny back surfaces of the upper and lower front teeth would possibly indicate an acid reflux problem. I check the shape and size of their tongue and look for recession of the gums. I look for scalloping along the sides of the tongue, check the size of their tonsils and the appearance of the uvula—is it elongated or does it look like normal size? If they have a lot of these factors, we feel pretty comfortable in saying that they may have an underlying sleep problem. As dentists, we often see these signs before the patient ever recognize that a problem exists. Patients often take medicine for various diseases or perhaps they take medicine to help them sleep, but they are only treating the symptoms. We need to treat the problem.

Every patient who presents with any kind of possibility of having sleep issues leaves our office with a home sleep screening device that we provide as a service. When they bring it back, we download the results of the test and will either refer them to a sleep physician or their Primary care physician for follow up. I can confidently say that we have saved lives because we've been able to take a patient who comes and says, "Yes, I don't sleep well," or maybe, "I'm just tired," and suggest a sleep screening. They might not even think to say anything to us, because we're dentists, and people don't always associate us with sleep issues. Interviewing our patients after they have been referred for their sleep study and been fitted with either a C-PAP, or fitted with and oral appliance at our office, all concede that the quality of their life has improved dramatically. Even to the point of being able to stay in the bedroom again with their spouse.

Here is an interesting story. One of my recent patients denied that he ever had any problems. He said, "There's no way that I have sleep problems. I do find that I may snore a little bit." We had him do a sleep screening at home, which indicated that he had sleep breathing issues. Next, we sent him to a sleep physician for a PSG (polysomnogram), which returned a value of 189 AHI (Apnea–Hypopnea Index, for which a normal value is 0–4). The sleep doctor said that he was surprised to find the patient still alive with that high of a number. He was fitted for a CPAP and when he came in our office for his hygiene visit, he said that he has never felt better. He has lost weight. He feels great all day and most importantly, his AHI has dropped to 3!

My goal is to continue to receive training to provide help for patients who cannot wear a continuous positive air pressure (CPAP) mask. The mask, which keeps air flowing through the airway during sleep, is the gold standard in the medical community for treating sleep apnea. Unfortunately, only about 30 percent of patients who need a CPAP will actually wear it. They do not like to wear a mask while they sleep. They might wear it occasionally in the beginning, but most of the time, they either take it off in the middle of the night or they just quit wearing it. Therefore, their sleep apnea is not being treated.

Oral appliances are approved for medical use to treat sleep apnea. They should only be provided by dentists trained in sleep medicine and dentistry as follow-up is essential for success. We can take care of these patients with a sleep appliance that is billed through their medical insurance. Patients must first be diagnosed by a sleep physician and give written consent that they are CPAP intolerant before they can be provided an oral appliance.

Someone once told me a really good summary of a dentist's work: "On a good day, we save a tooth. On a GREAT day, we save a life." We have done that by referring patients to their physicians, if they had high blood pressure during their dental visit. Besides sleep apnea screening, every person who arrives at our office as a new patient gets a blood pressure exam. We provide this as a standard service for all of our patients, even if they have no history of blood pressure problems. We are dentists AND we are physicians of the mouth. We are here to help our patients and lead them toward improving the health of their mouth and their body.

Quality sleep is truly the road to success regarding people's state of health. Untreated, sleep apnea can lead to a host of developmental, social, and behavioral problems throughout life. These problems tend to increase in their development over time, and a vast number of additional health problems rise exponentially when an apnea problem goes untreated. Ultimately, if left untreated, sleep apnea will result in premature death. As a general dentist, I feel that I am at the forefront of helping my patients live longer and healthier lives, improving their enjoyment and quality of life.

Sleep Apnea In Children

One of the other bits of information that has surprised many people is that children can also suffer from sleep apnea. Many parents do not realize that their child, whose breathing includes snoring, is suffering from a sleep disorder. *Snoring in children is not normal!*

Our body does its most important work while we sleep. In children, delta sleep or deep sleep accounts for 40 to 50 percent of sleep time. In adults, that drops down to about 10 to 25 percent of our total sleep. Children need delta sleep because that's when growth occurs. While this deep sleep goes on, the growth hormones reach their peak levels, and most body and cell recovery occurs at that time.

Until I started attending residency programs on this topic, I had no idea about the importance of sleep. People just take sleeping for granted because it is something that we all do. We sleep, and then we get up. If you wake up not feeling well or rested you just assume you had a bad night's sleep. Until you learn that all of this critical maintenance, repair, and recovery happens while you are sleeping, you don't really think about the importance of it.

Recently, a correlation between kids who have sleep disorder breathing and those who have ADHD has been found. The symptoms can be indistinguishable from each other, which can lead to misdiagnosis. Scientists have found that children who have any type of sleep disorder, including breathing (or snoring) issues, will tend to exhibit a number of alarming characteristics: childhood obesity, learning and behavioral issues, failure to thrive, and some hormonal and metabolic problems. These are also signs of ADHD. Obviously, this will negatively affect their growth and possibly their success as they get older. Children with ADHD can't concentrate on anything. They simply don't pay attention well, and they don't have good organizational skills. This is interesting: a child who doesn't sleep well usually exhibits similar symptoms and many of the same problems as one with ADHD. Children with destructive sleep apnea have increased rates of behavioral problems at home and at school, which negatively affects their learning and results in low academic performance. They also may be aggressive and unwilling to follow rules. (Think about your increased levels of intolerance that appear when you're tired.) The question then becomes this: are we treating for ADHD when we are actually dealing with poor sleep?

When a child reaches adulthood, if they are still being treated for ADHD, and labeled as such, they may display the common symptoms of sleep disorder breathing that create difficulties in concentrating and completing tasks. They may also show poor skill levels and memory lapses that will impact their success as adults.

It's terribly important—critical, in fact—to have dentists who are on the leading edge of sleep apnea in children, examine children at age one and two for certain signs. We need to check their tonsils, see their growth patterns, and see if they have a recessed jaw. We also need to check for tongue tie as this also affects the development of infants. We can guide parents into being proactive and seeking treatment at a very young and developmental age and not waiting until the signs lead to the problems.

This is a good example. I started coming back from these learning events, excited about all of this new information. I shared some of what I had learned with my associate whose daughter had needed to get tubes placed into her ears. "Jill, you've got to have this doctor look at her tonsils and her adenoids."

Jill did have this checked out because her daughter had all of the symptoms: she didn't sleep well and was restless and rambunctious during the day. She had the child's tonsils taken out and the adenoids removed. The doctor said they were the biggest adenoids that he had ever seen in a child that age. This intervention improved the quality of both of their lives—a mother can sleep better because her daughter's sleeping better. This is just one of those success stories that I could tell. It simply involves educating parents about healthy and unhealthy patterns: "It's not normal for your child to snore. It's not normal for children to grind their teeth. They may be grinding their teeth because they are trying to open their airway. Bedwetting and frequent nightmares are also early signs of sleep disorder breathing."

There is a great number of commonly occurring incidents that people are just not paying attention to. For that matter, physicians aren't paying attention, either. They just say, "We're going to put you on Ritalin." That's just treating the symptom and not addressing the underlying problem.

We're able to look in a child's mouth and see if the mouth is too small to accommodate the tongue or if the lower jaw is too short or recessed. Those conditions will cause a child's tongue to fall back so that he or she has to struggle to breathe at night. If he sees this issue, the pediatric dentist will basically say, "We need to get this kid started with an orthodontist soon."

As dentists, we have the advantage of being able to help the jaw develop better than it would without help. With orthodontic appliances, we're able to correct cross-bites, which expand the upper jaw and make more room for the tongue. We're able to see changes in facial patterns. The kids who have difficulty in breathing often have long faces and breathe through their mouths because their jaws are too small for them to take proper breaths. By getting the young ones to an orthodontist or general dentist early, their jaws can be properly developed employing orthopedic appliances while they are still in the developmental stage.

Two of my patients were referred to me as children because they had sleep apnea and wouldn't wear a CPAP device. Children can wear CPAPs, but they don't like it any more than adults do, so they resist wearing it. We were able to get them in an oral appliance to treat their sleep apnea with success.

I expect that many children showing these symptoms are not being treated for sleep apnea. They are being treated for hyperactivity and—this is what's so important—they are being misdiagnosed. Doctors, dentists, and especially parents need to know that many of these symptoms are sleep-related. Bed-wetting is a classic sign and so is snoring. It isn't a normal facet of childhood life; it's related to sleep disorder breathing. Parents often don't know that because pediatricians also don't know that, and it's alarming!

When professionals from our office go to these classes to learn more about this problem, we hear ear, nose, and throat (ENT) specialists saying, "We get a one-hour lecture, or maybe one full day of lectures, on the topic of sleep apnea in medical school." That's really sad if you consider the risks associated with sleep disorders.

I think it's so important for dentists to look at the tonsils and adenoids and refer the patient to the ENT specialist for removal. In itself, that surgery has been shown to eliminate sleep apnea in 79 percent of the children who go through the surgery. By checking for signs of grinding on baby teeth in their first permanent molars, along with behavioral problems (chronic bed wetting, bad dreams, snoring), there's a good probability that the specialist is seeing signs of obstructive sleep apnea. Even chronic ear infections and tubes suggest that there could be a poorly developed upper jaw. There's a great deal of overlap between dentistry and other branches of medicine. It's great that we're able to bridge some of those gaps.

The Future Of Dentistry

If you don't get on the bandwagon of the future, as a dentist, you will be left behind. It's no longer just graduating from dental school and opening up a dental practice anymore. Dentists have to be willing to invest time in learning other parts of our profession. Learn more about sedation dentistry. Learn to use the available technology so that you don't have to send out to someone else to create the crown. Keep up with the technology, use it, and bring it into your practice.

For instance, we've had a CEREC machine since the year 2000 (the system that we use for creating individual all-ceramic restorations in a single appointment); it was sold through Patterson Dental. It was a beast when you tried to design anything. We had to use powder; it was just a mess, besides the hassle of the steep learning curve. My assistant got sick, so we had to put the training on the back burner, and every new associate resisted getting trained on the machine, because they thought, "it's not the future." When my son joined the practice in 2012, on his first day, I said, "Okay, you're going to get training on how to use the CEREC." Within a year, he is now a trainer and a mentor. We have three Omnicams and a Bluecam for our offices. And 90% of our crowns are now done in the office. This technology has reduced overhead and has been an excellent marketing tool as well. Patients love the idea of getting their crown the same day.

Another big element of a dental practice is cosmetic dentistry. That's a field that is all about art and keeping up with the technology. There is no officially recognized specialty called "cosmetic dentistry". We are all general dentists, but extra training is available. Most of us do a passable job at creating a beautiful, more aesthetic smile, but there is no replacement for a dentist that specializes in this field of dentistry. They have done the additional training and are more artful in what they do, because cosmetic dentistry is, honestly, an art form. To do it well, dentists need to concentrate their education on cosmetic work and get all of the extra training that they can to build their skill levels and be able to comfortably say that they can provide cosmetic services to their patients.

I consider myself a comprehensive dentist able to provide care in all facets of dentistry with emphasis on cosmetics. We evaluate every patient for optimal health as well as optimal comfort and aesthetics. Often full mouth reconstruction must be done to improve function as well as aesthetics. Patients improve their self-esteem, their ability to get a job, their relationships. It's rewarding to take patients from not wanting to smile to being comfortable when they smile; it's rewarding to provide an improvement in their viewpoint of how they feel about themselves. We provide our services in a relaxing and comfortable environment and make it affordable and an investment that will last a lifetime.

As a dentist for the next generation, you also have to be innovative in every way. You need to discover and implement the things that make patients want to come back. A lot of people don't like visiting dentists, and I am one of them. Quite simply, my experience was a bad experience. I elected not to have my fillings done with anesthetic. It was the most horrible thing that I've ever done. I hear similar stories from other patients, that they've had a bad experience—somebody hurt them, or the dentist didn't care that the procedure was hurting them and he kept drilling, even though they tried to get him to stop.

When I see these patients who are scared, there's always a story about something that happened when they were kids that instilled that fear in them. Certainly, because of my bad experience, I can empathize with them right away and just say, "This is why we do what we do here."

In our office, we provide massage therapists to come and massage patients' hands and arms while they're either in the hygiene room or in the treatment room with us. We also have warm paraffin wax for their hands. Patients will say that it's the best thing that's ever happened because it just works like magic to take away that anxiety that they're feeling when they're here.

Of course, just as most dental offices do, we also provide nitrous oxide. We have the headsets, which most offices do these days. We use warm paraffin wax and give blankets to our patients. We have a coffee bar with fresh-made cookies every day. We do a number of things to change the usual aesthetic of the "dentist's office", and to take away the sterile feel.

All of these little amenities are distinctive; they set us apart, I think, because a lot of offices don't have them. It also makes the patients so much more comfortable when they walk in. Also, our offices don't look like dental offices. They look like living rooms. They don't smell like dental offices—at least, I hope they don't.

We hope that our offices smell like fresh coffee and cookies. Baking bread is an excellent way to mask the smell of a dental office, as well. Just watch out! It's hard to resist eating it yourself!

We also experiment. Through the grapevine in Lexington, I've heard that some people just can't believe that I offer cookies to my patients because they just promote tooth decay. Here's my opinion: we have to think outside the box. We have to stand in the patient's shoes. We can't always think like dentists if we are going to relate to the patients. I've always been more risk-taking in the sense that I want to know the patients' perception and how it makes them feel. There are some things that we've done, marketing-wise, that just didn't work. So, we try something else until we find something that makes our patients say, "I really appreciate the fact that you do that."

To make our anxious patients feel better, we do both oral sedation and also IV sedation. Those options are available for patients who have anxiety. We don't actually provide Valium, but they can take Valium. That's a very nice way to just take off the edge. The lowest level of a sedation option for a nervous patient—it works quite well—is a Valium an hour before the dental visit. It works for the patient to take five milligrams an hour before he arrives at the office and gets put on nitrous oxide. That works for the majority of patients. Nitrous oxide, by itself, works pretty well. I usually use that if the patient says, "I'm a little bit nervous about this," but not to the anxiety level where they need something just to get to sleep on the night before the procedure.

We also do the oral sedation method. This means that the patient takes the pill right before coming into the dental office, and remains sleepy throughout the visit. Most patients don't even remember the visit. The same is true with IV sedation, which my son does for us right now. It's a little bit deeper sedation than oral sedation, but very, very safe. All of these options are very safe. Every patient gets monitored with a pulse oximeter. We make sure that we watch their blood pressure, oxygen levels, and so on throughout the process. You can get all of your dentistry done in one visit and there are no bad memories.

It's important to know that not all dentists have these options readily available in order to take care of anxious patients. First, some fairly serious certification has to happen. A dentist must get one or more certifications, specific trainings for a specific amount of hours, and listen to many lectures—things like that. My son, Ryan, took some of these specific IV sedation courses at dental school last year—four weekends of intensive training.

After the dentist gets the specialized training, it's necessary to apply for the license through the Kentucky Board of Industry. It's also necessary to have a special certification and a license to do oral sedation, which is the method that I use. Dentists can't do sedation without this license. As a patient, if you have anxiety issues, ask about sedation options as you make that first appointment.

As I get ready to plan for retirement, I plan and strive toward getting into sleep apnea and/or the dentist's role in sleep apnea. That is my passion. I plan to further my education beyond what I've already done. I have attended Tufts in Boston, I've done mini-residencies in dental and medical sleep medicine, and I will continue to pursue knowledge about this problem as I move forward. With both of my children taking on more tasks and responsibility in the offices, I'll also be able to spend more time strengthening our business network among medical doctors and dentists. This is where the future of health care is going: toward more of a focus on care and maintenance of the whole body.

(This content should be used for informational purposes only. It does not create a doctor-patient relationship with any reader and should not be construed as medical advice. If you need medical advice, please contact a doctor in your community who can assess the specifics of your situation.)

7

Find Your Passion, Your Life's Purpose And Go After It With Zeal, Tenacity, And Joy!

by Terri Baarstad, D.M.D.

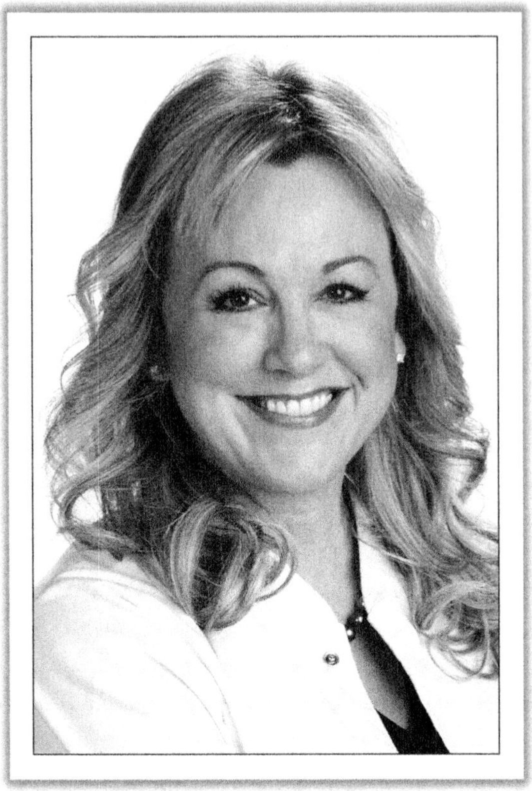

Terri Baarstad, D.M.D.

SmileAlive
Eugene, Oregon
www.smilealive.com

Dr. Terri Baarstad, the owner and practicing dentist at SmileAlive is known for her pleasant manner and down-to-earth personality. She has a knack for "putting herself in her patients' shoes", and being sensitive to their comfort level. Under Dr. Baarstad's care, you can be confident that her consultation will be with your best interest at heart.

Along with her Husband and children, Dr. Baarstad has made Eugene her home for over 30 years. She enjoys spending time with family, friends, and her dogs. Her hobbies include fishing, scuba diving, photography and cooking.

Dr. Baarstad appreciates the value of community service, and devotes herself to improving the dental health of those who live around her. She donates services to charitable organizations and sponsors many community events, including high school fundraisers. Dr. Baarstad expresses a special interest in helping young men and women explore a career in dentistry through volunteering at local high school career symposiums.

After attending the University of Oregon, Dr. Baarstad graduated as a DMD from the Oregon Health Sciences University in Portland. She is an active member of the American Dental Association, the Oregon Dental Association, and the Academy of General Dentistry, and a recipient of the Dr. William Howard Award for Excellence in Fixed Prosthetics. She is especially skilled in the areas of dental implants, cosmetic care, including crowns and bridges, porcelain veneers, traditional and implant dentures. Her experience is enriched by a focus on continuing education, including courses on comprehensive esthetics and implantology.

Find Your Passion, Your Life's Purpose And Go After It With Zeal, Tenacity, And Joy!

A Little Bit About My Childhood

I am the fourth of six children. My mother was 23 years old when I was born. I grew up relatively poor in an old farmhouse in West Salem. It is suburbia now, but it was rural when I was a kid. Our nearest neighbor was about a half- mile down the road, and our home was surrounded by cherry orchards, wheat fields, honey trees, big oaks and plenty of fresh air. It wasn't exactly a farm, but we had a giant vegetable garden, chickens, and plenty of dogs and cats. We even had the occasional baby quail, pheasant or Guinea pig brought home from school for the summer. Our playground consisted of dirt roads, trails through wheat fields, and the ponds and streams that flowed through the property. My father hunted and fished so we had fresh meats, and we grew or gleaned whatever else we ate. What wasn't eaten right away was canned or frozen for later. My grandmother hand-ground her wheat into flour, not the norm for the 1970's.

My mother was a young, somewhat naive, but loving mom. She was strict and religious, expecting us to do our chores, and homework, and to generally behave ourselves. My parents divorced when I was 7, and I didn't see my father frequently after that. To be honest, we didn't see him much before the divorce. To be kind, he was not an admirable man. He definitely did not make his family a priority. I was a happy, easy, middle child amongst fairly rowdy, aggressive, risk-taking siblings. I was the good kid. I never got into trouble, and I earned good grades, so that generally guaranteed my invisibility.

My mom married again, when I was 12, and we moved to Eugene. My step dad was a good provider. My mother was able to quit working so hard and relax a little, and our lifestyle was more comfortable, which was a nice change. I had not really comprehended how hard it had been on my mother. I went to North Eugene High School and graduated in 1985. Education had never been a priority in my family. I was the first person in my family to graduate with my class. Because no one had yet negotiated the world of college, applications and financial aid, it seemed a little daunting to consider going to college, but I was determined. I had some great teachers who encouraged and helped me tremendously. Never underestimate your power to influence someone's life.

Influential Things From My Childhood: Frogs, Salamanders And Grandpa Riley

As I look back at my childhood and think about what made me happy, I realize that it was exploring the outdoors. I loved being with my dog, checking out the frogs and salamanders living in the creek, the trees that housed the honeycombs, the Native American artifacts, and old coins we discovered, digging around the property. I was always very curious. While my family situation was not ideal, I was happy and felt loved.

If I had to choose someone who influenced me while I was growing up, it would be my grandparents. They were hardworking, kind people who loved their grandchildren. We would take turns having sleepovers at their small, modest home in Rickreall, Oregon. My grandfather would take us on long walks. Often, we would stop by the old store with its creaky wooden floors, where we could choose a pack of Wrigley's spearmint gum and two boxes of cracker Jacks. Walking side by side, we would eat the cracker jacks down the abandoned tracks, my five year old legs stretching to hit the railroad ties. I always hoped to get the stick-on tattoos as my Cracker Jack prize. Strangely, Grandpa always managed to find them in his box. I would bargain for a trade, and he would swap whatever inferior prize I had, and then help me ink my freckled arms. He passed away when I was 5. It's funny, but when my siblings and I get together, it is a well known fact who was whose "favorite child".

"You were Grandma's favorite. You were Dad's favorite. You were Mom's favorite." But all six of us are convinced that we were Grandpa Riley's favorite. He had the gift of making you feel special and important.

My College Education

I attended the University of Oregon, majoring in Chemistry/ pre-med. Within the first year, I got very sick, earned the first C of my lifetime, became engaged, and ran out of money. I didn't understand financial aid or scholarships, and I couldn't work enough hours to cover tuition costs. Discouraged, I quit going to University and went to Lane Community College. I searched through the programs at the community college and decided to become a dental assistant. The program was nine months long and relatively inexpensive, and I could earn enough money to start a family.

I was 19 when I began working as a dental assistant. Within a year of working in the dental field and observing my boss, a great dentist, I told myself "You could do what he's doing." It would be another 10 years before I enrolled in dental school. During that time, I observed and learned about the profession. When I was working, I would ask Dr. Laing, "Why do you do this? What happens with that? Why does that tooth fail and that one does not?" I was very curious about how things worked and why the dentists would choose to do various procedures over other procedures. I thought dentistry was fascinating and interesting, very mechanical but very artistic. Life circumstances didn't allow me to return to school for a long time. I had two small children, an unhappy husband and a relatively low paying job. When I got divorced, I knew I couldn't support my children by myself on a dental assistant's income. More importantly, I felt that I hadn't reached my potential. My inner voice was telling me, "There's more for you to do." That is when I decided to go to Oregon Health Sciences University to become a dentist.

Typically, it takes four to five years to complete the prerequisites required for application to dental school. Most people receive a college degree and then apply to dental school. Because I was a single mother of two, I was in a hurry to complete my education and start my practice. I researched the necessary requirements for dental school and began taking the classes: Core Biology, Core Chemistry, Organic chemistry, Physics - all of which were yearlong courses- each term following the next. I needed four terms of math classes to meet the requirements for these core classes, which would set me back a year or two. Therefore, I begged my instructors to allow me to enter their classes without the appropriate prerequisites and they agreed, as long as I didn't ask them any math questions.

I enrolled into the Core Chemistry classes at Lane Community College and made my first epic mistake. Unknowingly, I entered the yearlong Chemistry course for NON- health-care professionals. That series would definitely not fulfill my requirements for dental school. I discovered this problem only two weeks prior to the end of the term. I would have to wait until the next fall, 9 months later, to take the correct course series. I was devastated. My instructor took pity on me and set up a meeting with the other instructor, and we devised a plan. I would self-study the first term, taking all the exams and the final exam in the next two weeks, in addition to completing the other three courses I was currently taking, and working 35 hours a week while being a single mom. Only then would I qualify to take the remainder of the series and stay on track. And, did I mention, I needed an A for the grade. It took me three years to complete my pre-dental education. I was working as a dental assistant approximately 36-40 hours a week to support my children. I went to school at night the first year and a half at the community college, and then I transferred to the university. I also did a term of summer school. I don't know if you've ever taken summer school, but for me, that summer was very intense. As I was walking to my final in Physics, I remember thinking this is what it feels like to be pushed to the edge of my limits.

During this time, I had virtually no support system. In fact, all of my friends, (save one, my friend Peggy) my family, the man I was dating, and my boss all told me I was crazy - there was no way I could do this. They said I needed to be realistic and set my sights on hygiene or sales, something less demanding. I didn't want to do either of those. Being a dentist was my calling.

Owning My Power & Realizing My Self-Worth

An event that had a great influence on me was a group of courses put on by PSI Seminars. My mother and sister asked me to go, telling me I would get to know myself better and become more successful. I wasn't interested. I had a busy dental practice, a new husband, my two children, and three stepchildren to raise. My mom asked me to trust her and just go, and although it was a tough sell, I went. "Have an open mind" was her advice. I spent seven days with strangers doing exercises designed to help you evaluate your thought process and your belief system to see if they are serving you the best way in your life. They also make you uncomfortable. At these courses, I came to understand things about myself that weren't helping me. I recognized habits, beliefs and self-talk that were preventing me from being my own best advocate. A particularly difficult event for me was climbing a wobbly, telephone-sized pole. I had been dreading this exercise for over a year. I was petrified of heights. While I was in no real danger because I was in a harness and had redundant safety features in place, it did not matter to my brain. Just prior to my ascent, the coach took me aside and said to me, "You've been trying to prove your whole life that you're worthy. You can't really prove that. It's something you just believe. For example, if you're a person who believes in God, you don't try to prove that God exists. You just believe that He does."

One of the activities was a very challenging group ropes course. We were tired, hot, cranky and hungry at the end of a long day when the leaders told us we had one more challenge. No one was happy about it. The exercise involved a very complex physical feat, one that required planning, delicate execution, and full co-operation of the entire 26-person team to succeed. Under the best of circumstances it looked improbable. To make things even more challenging, we were not allowed to speak. After some various unsuccessful attempts, I began to take charge with hand signals. With the help of another teammate, we were able to accomplish the giant task in record time. The course was life-changing for me as I emerged from that experience as a well-liked and well-respected leader. The facilitator came to me later that night to congratulate me as the first female leader in the history of this exercise.

Those experiences empowered me and helped me realize that I had many gifts and inner strength. I was able to recognize and celebrate all of the things that I had accomplished. I was able to accept that my thoughts, feelings, needs and wants were important. It may sound self-evident, but it was an epiphany for me and a major turning point in my life.

In our society, valuable things aren't ignored. My childhood family structure was not healthy. As the quiet "middle-child" and the peacemaker, I never really learned that my wants and needs mattered. To some degree, my marriages were a continuation of that. If your father, the one man who should adore you and keep you safe, abandons you and your family, it affects you on a deep level. If you don't fix those hurt feelings, those insecurities stay with you. As a child, you adopt messages, interpret them, and then you begin to believe the "lies we tell ourselves". Many people are riddled on some deep level with the fear of not feeling worthy of being loved or respected. I read recently that even highly successful Fortune 500 CFOs and CEOs have this deep-down fear that they'll be found out for not being as "important" as they appear.

My friend Kris explains not everyone feels this way. "I've never felt like I had to be perfect or that I wasn't worthy of being loved." However, I have another friend, 35 years old, who was raised in the same type of healthy family environment with structure and morals, love and attention, and yet he struggles daily with self-doubt and worry. I don't know what causes that for one person and not for another. Our value isn't based on media, what our parents did or didn't do, or the mistakes we've made. It is OK to not be perfect. When you tell yourself, "I'm worthless. My life is ruined," you are telling yourself lies. If you're going to lie to yourself, make it a good lie." Say, "I'm the most amazing person in the whole world."

There is a great book out right now, called Positive Intelligence, by Chamine, that addresses this thinking. The voices in our head always work for or against us. Harness that, control your self-talk and make it work for you. As a woman in my 40's, my perceptions about myself and my self-talk have changed.

Thankfully, I've become more reality-based, kinder and gentler. I sometimes hear a young woman say that she has gained five pounds and she's "disgusting". I remember feeling this way. Fortunately, as I have matured if I gain five pounds, I don't think I'm disgusting. I just think, "I need to take these five pounds off."

Our society is hard on women. In addition to dealing with blatant sexism and inequality in the workforce, we are supposed to be beautiful, smart, sexy, successful business people, devoted mothers, and creative artists. That is a lot of pressure. There's a sense that if you're not perfect, then you're not worthy. The reality is that none of us is perfect and yet we're all worthy. We are just all a little bit broken in some way. Remembering this when dealing with ourselves and others is the key to being compassionate.

The Best Decisions I Made

There are three "Best Decision I Ever Made" events in my life: having children, becoming a dentist, and marrying Jim. My life now is incredible. Jim is an amazing husband and our marriage is very supportive, nurturing and stable. I have peace. He is respectful, kind, and intelligent, and he treats me well. Our children are doing well. Two of our children are married, and they chose good partners. I encourage my children to live with integrity and make decisions that they believe are the right ones. I believe you should be your own friend, encourage yourself, believe in yourself, and be kind to yourself.

I tell my family and friends that my life is perfect, "right now". I am appreciating all the blessings I have. I know nothing is "perfect" and that at any moment lives can change, but I am sure enjoying this time in my life. This makes being successful as a dentist a lot easier. I wouldn't say it's easy, but I love my job, and it's a lot easier because I have support. I have 13 incredible women on my staff, two of whom have been with me for more than 10 years. They are amazing. As well as being smart, ambitious, and virtuous, they are loyal and they are my friends. As a business owner, I would say hire smart people, train them and get out of their way. They will make your life a lot easier. Don't forget to treat them accordingly.

My Philosophy Of Dentistry And The Care That I Provide To My Patients

My philosophy for patient care is that there are three main categories of dentistry: Treating Disease, Restoring Form and Function, and Aesthetics. Treating disease is "doctor-driven", meaning that I will push a patient a little bit in this arena, because I will lose sleep if patients don't achieve health. Diseases of the mouth, not including oral cancer, come from two basic sources, gum disease and tooth decay. The most important thing to me is that my patients are disease-free. How you treat the disease and the level of treatment to be performed is dependent on the needs and desires of that patient; however, the goal is the same for everyone — to be disease-free.

The second phase of dentistry is Restoring Form and Function. If you have a broken tooth, it needs to be repaired. If you are missing teeth and have reduced function, you need to replace teeth. If you need braces, a night-guard, or have failing restorations, there are solutions. This second phase of dentistry is really about restoring the "chewing machine" and moving the patient closer to ideal. This is more patient-driven. I make sure that my patients are educated about conditions they could improve, the options for treatment, the costs, and long term pros and cons. I answer all their questions.

The third phase is aesthetics, which is patient-driven. Again, I will educate patients about their options, but I do not push cosmetic dentistry. It depends on the desires of that patient. Every person's idea of aesthetics is different. In America we value a beautiful, straight, white smile. I don't think everyone needs braces and whitening. I do believe you need to be able to smile freely, without reservation or embarrassment to be truly healthy. For some, when they achieve a healthy confident smile, it will be life changing. I have seen it happen and it is one of the best parts of my job.

There are times when we can fix all three things with one solution. If you have a cavity on the front tooth, we will make it aesthetically pleasing, restore the function of the tooth, and treat the disease all at once. In some cases, we can phase things out over a period of time to help the patient financially afford to do everything needed to treat the disease, restore function, and have an attractive, confident smile.

THE FUTURE OF DENTISTRY

We have CAD/CAM dentistry, which allows us to do many things. We make digital replications of the entire head and neck, examine various structures, even pre-plan size and locations of implants. We take digital impressions. We use a 3D camera that captures an image of your entire mouth in great detail. We use that image to make Invisalign®- type braces, fabricate crowns, onlays and bridgework, or make study models. Instead of taking a traditional impression, then pouring in stone and making a casting from that, we can take the digital image, send it wirelessly to a printer and it prints out a model. It is more accurate, quicker, and has the advantage of not using the "gooey stuff" that patients tend not to like.

Digital x-rays are another amazing advancement in dentistry. They require a tiny fraction of the radiation compared to medical radiographs (x-rays). There are no chemicals needed to develop them, and they simply pop up on our screen within seconds. We take a CAT scan of the head to determine exactly where vital structures are to create computer-assisted surgical guides, allowing us to place dental implants exactly where they need to be for the best outcome.

In my offices, we have a CEREC, which is a CAD/cam machine. We prep the tooth for a crown and then we image it. We have a milling unit that uses diamond burs to cut out the crown from dilithium-silicate block. It is called e.max®. When it comes out of the milling machine, it is lavender. Our patient bibs happen to be that exact color, so I tease the patients that I just LOVE that color so much we make EVERYTHING lavender. The crown fits the tooth perfectly. We custom stain and glaze it, put it into the ceramic firing oven and fire right there in our office. Because we can do this in our office in one session, the patient never has to wear a temporary crown or have gooey impressions. People are amazed by these advances. They love to watch me design the crown and then go out to the waiting room to watch the crown appear out of a solid block. The milling unit is in the waiting room so the patients can watch the process.

Baby boomers don't want removable appliances in their mouths. They do want aesthetically attractive, fully functioning chewing machines until they die. Today, we have many dental options that are painless and relatively quick. And, the restorations are more aesthetic and last longer. We just added a Dental Vibe in our office. We place a vibrating hand-held device next to the area to be anesthetized. When the needle is slipped delicately into the tissue, the patient doesn't feel a thing. It works on the gateway theory that our nerves can only transmit one sensation. Our patients love it and frequently ask, "Does that vibrating thing just numb me up or are you still going to give me a shot?" I tell them, "I already gave you the shot." It is absolutely amazing. Typically, when you numb the front of the mouth, under the nose or in the palate, it can be unpleasant, because there are so many nerve endings in the area. The palate is also uncomfortable because there's no room for the fluid to go into that area, and it is almost impossible to give a truly painless injection. With the Dental Vibe, the patients say, "Oh my gosh! I didn't feel anything!" It is very satisfying when you can give an injection and the patient literally doesn't know that you just did it.

DENTISTRY AND OVERALL PERSONAL HEALTHCARE

Today, we know that what happens in the mouth is connected to the body. For a long time, people would say, "I take really, really good care of myself. I'm a runner and an athlete. I only eat organic foods. Sure, I have a few cavities, but that's not big deal. I have gum disease, but that's no big deal either." We know that if you have gum disease, or you have cavities that are significant, you might lose a tooth. It's more than just losing your teeth. You may not consider that to be too serious. However, if you constantly have low-grade chronic infection in your body, particularly if you have an immune-compromised system, like people with diabetes or arthritis, this low-grade chronic infection changes your blood chemistry and makes you more prone to disease. Countless studies show that inflammation is key to creating a diseased body. If we can reduce the amount of inflammation in our bodies, particularly in our mouths, then overall we're healthier.

People don't see their family doctor as often as they see their dentist. We screen all of our patients for blood pressure, thyroid issues, oral cancer and head and neck/ skin cancers. Often, you'll discover a blood pressure issue when you're at the dentist. Some people have elevated blood pressure because they are nervous about being at the dentist. However, if their blood pressure has been elevated the last few times they have been at the dental office or if their pressure is significantly high, we will refer them to their family doctor to have that checked out. If necessary, we facilitate a patient getting to the emergency room or the urgent care when the medical condition warrants that immediate attention.

If you're a smoker or a person who chews tobacco, it is especially important that we do a cancer screening at every visit. We also look down the throat for acid reflux or GERD. We look for enlarged tonsils and nodes on the back of the throat. Patients may not even have any symptoms but as dentists, we can detect medical concerns during our exam so the patient can seek early treatment.

Sleep apnea is another issue that dentists treat. It's a huge problem in America, partly because so many Americans are overweight, but there are many causes. Consider holding your breath 100 times a night, every night. Your body is starving for oxygen, and it puts a huge strain on your body, especially the heart. People with sleep apnea have a tendency to clench their teeth when they sleep. We can make assessments based on what the teeth look like, what the airway is like and other oral signs.

The wear patterns on your teeth often tell another story. Dentists are likely to notice when a patient is bulimic, because there is an erosion pattern that is very distinctive to repeated vomiting. We can discover arthritis of the jaw joints, calcification of the carotid arteries, and other conditions because they show up on our radiographic exams.

We don't think about people dying from a toothache, but it can happen. Overuse and misuse of antibiotics have created resistant strains of bacteria that make some infections impossible to cure. Realize that our upper teeth are close to our brain, and that infection in our lower teeth can travel down the vertebral column and infect the heart. It is very rare, but it is tragic when it happens. Take antibiotics exactly as your doctor prescribes them. It is also important for your dentist to know all your medical conditions and medications, because they affect how you may heal, complications that may arise, and how we may best treat you.

There are many ways that dentists participate in overall health. For example, diabetic patients need to have their teeth cleaned more often, approximately every 3 months. Gum disease can affect diabetes and vice versa. When someone is diagnosed with cancer, particularly if they will be receiving radiation, it's vitally important we see them for a thorough examination to anticipate any oral complications from chemo and/or radiation. If they have teeth that are diseased, these teeth often need to be removed prior to radiation. Once a jaw has been radiated it's impossible to extract teeth without risk of severe complications. We also work with orthopedic and cardiac surgeons to ensure patients understand the importance of dental health prior to knee or valve replacement surgeries. Pre-medication may be prescribed before a teeth cleaning appointment to avoid complications of bacteria infecting the heart, hip or knee. These are severe complications that can be life-threatening. Health risks are much higher when oral health has not been maintained. Guidelines have changed frequently over the last few years so make sure your dentist and doctor are keeping abreast of these recommendations.

Dealing With Dental Fears

I had a filling done today by my associate dentist. I used the "Dental Vibe" to anesthetize the area and felt nothing except the onset of numbness. I plugged in my headphones, turned up John Mayer and tuned out. I call it "empathy training" because it helps me to understand how my patients feel. Lying back with one's mouth propped open, you are in a vulnerable position that can be stressful even for me the patient/doctor. This time I felt completely relaxed. Why? It occurred to me that I trusted Dr. Kevin 100%, and I was completely numb - 2 essential components of a good dental experience. The message I want to send to patients is to find a dentist you trust completely. Interview potential dentists if necessary. I want to have a positive relationship with our patients so that I can treat them holistically for a lifetime. At SmileAlive, we believe that going to the dentist should not be scary.

We joke in our office that dentistry is never going to be dinner and dancing. It's never going to be a trip to Disneyland, but it shouldn't be scary. It should not be painful. There may be procedures that have some post-operative discomfort, but we can manage that discomfort. If you have fears that are rational or irrational, it doesn't matter, we can manage those too. There are ways to work through the fear so that you can be healthy. We offer medications, blankets, headphones, pillows and comfort. Communicate with your providers — we really do want your experience to be as pleasant as possible. We want to provide excellent customer service. If you don't feel like you are getting this level of service from your dentist, then you're not in the right place.

In Closing

Life is grand. As my mother said, "Life is full of character-building experiences." It's not what happens to you as much as how you respond to those events. Find your passion, your life's purpose and go after it with zeal, tenacity and joy. My other advice to women in particular - Don't limit yourself or your dreams. I hear young women say they want to be a dental hygienist or a nurse, and my question is always, "Why not the doctor?" If your goal is to be a nurse - wonderful. For some women, however, becoming the doctor is too big a dream, too much school, too much money, too much time, "I'll be too old." There was a time when I wondered whether becoming a dentist might be out of reach. Today, I can tell you to dream big, make the commitment, work hard and go for it. If I can do it, so can you.

(This content should be used for informational purposes only. It does not create a doctor-patient relationship with any reader and should not be construed as medical advice. If you need medical advice, please contact a doctor in your community who can assess the specifics of your situation.)

8

The Importance Of Proper Dental Care From Toddlers Through Adults

by Trevor Tsuchikawa D.D.S.

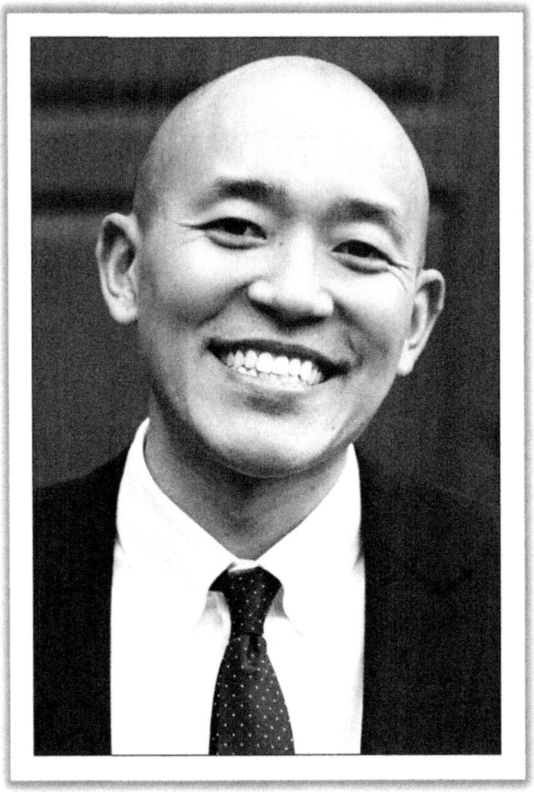

Trevor Tsuchikawa D.D.S.
Dr. Trevor Family Dentistry
Seattle, Washington
www.drtrevordentistry.com

Dr. Trevor Tsuchikawa practices dentistry in the community he was born and raised. He takes extreme pride in understanding people and their individual concerns. Dr. Trevor graduated from Seattle University where he majored in Biochemistry and played on the basketball team. He then received his Doctorate of Dental Surgery from the University of Washington, School of Dentistry.

Dr. Trevor is a major sports fan and was a proud member of the basketball coaching staff at his alma mater Franklin High School. Dr. Trevor and his wife Marisa have two beautiful daughters Taylor and Tanna. They are the drive of his life and he takes as much pride in fatherhood as anyone. Some of his hobbies include basketball, soccer, personal development, traveling, and experiencing life with his friends and family.

Through a combination of state of the art technology, sensible treatment plans and genuine devotion to the unique needs of each patient, Dr. Trevor has been honored as one of "America's Top Dentist" by Consumer Research. Applying unique blend of artistic and technical skills to produce durable and aesthetic results in thousands of patients. Dr. Trevor is dedicated to lifelong learning through continuing education courses. He is licensed by the Dental Board of Washington and is a member of the American Dental Association, Washington State Dental Association, King County Dental Society, and American Academy of General Dentistry. He is also a proud member of Sunrise Dental and attributes nearly all of his success as a dentist to his mentors Dr. Edward Im and Dr. Abraham Ghorbanian.

THE IMPORTANCE OF PROPER DENTAL CARE FROM TODDLERSTHROUGH ADULTS

A LITTLE BIT ABOUT MY BACKGROND

I was born and raised in Seattle, Washington. It's a wonderful place to live and grow up, and I'm a very proud Seattleite. I lived in the inner city part of Seattle and grew up around trouble in the neighborhood and in school. My family kept me motivated and ambitious. My family has been extremely influential in my life. We weren't the stereotypical Asian family, but my parents were very hard workers who were very serious about instilling good values of hard work in my brother and me. They were very hard-working people, and I like to think that I am as dedicated as they taught me to be.

I grew up with one younger brother, whom I spent every day with and don't know what I would do without the guy. My parents saw the value of athletics in teaching young people discipline and focus, so they kept me involved in a lot of sports. I thought I was on track to be the first Asian in the NBA. I played soccer, baseball, and basketball; all of these activities kept me pretty busy. I learned so much thru sports and played basketball at Franklin High School and also at Seattle University. Being a 5'7" Asian kid trying to play college basketball definitely made me tougher. Sports is a different world and you see people's true drive in sports.

I majored in Biochemistry and then went on to study dentistry at the University of Washington. I fell in love with the profession and the way that a dentist can diagnose and treat the patient on the spot. I knew that I wanted to run my own dental office, and the profession seemed like a much better fit for my dreams and ambitions. So that was the career choice that I made, and I'm very happy with it.

A few events have really influenced my life. One in particular had a huge impact on me—I suffered a stroke about eight years ago. Such an event has a way of teaching you that life is short. When you have a brush with mortality, it helps you prioritize your day-to-day life; you realize that it's necessary to appreciate what you have, enjoy the people around you, and spend the time that you have doing what matters most to you. I still live by that rule, even though I'm now fully recovered and have suffered no residual effects from the stroke. I still appreciate everything that I have, and of course I'm still striving for more, but I try not to clutter up my life with meaningless things.

Suffering a stroke can be extremely humbling, but it also taught me a lot about myself. It showed me that your will and drive can define who you are. I was so driven that I wasn't going to let this stroke stop me. Nor was I going to let this define me or my life story. I didn't feel sorry for myself and got back on the horse. I couldn't wait to continue on my chosen path.

Another major impact in my life was the birth of my first child. I am married to my high school sweetheart, Marisa, and we have two beautiful children: Taylor and Tanna. My children became my reason for doing a lot of things. In my case, my sense of motivation and ambition really shot through the roof once the kids came along. Naturally, as a parent, you want what's best for them. I wanted to provide my children with the best and want to be able to provide the most opportunities for them. They are my "why". Everyone has a "why" for waking up in the morning or wanting to achieve something. Never forgetting my "why" drives me every day.

Also, as a parent, you want to be free to spend as much time as possible with your kids. You take all of the necessary steps in order to provide everything for them to be safe, happy, and healthy. I read and listen to as much material as I can on improving myself so I can be the best person I can be for them. As you can see, I take the business of raising children very seriously.

Another life-changing event for me was the process of joining Sunrise Dental. That association has provided numerous opportunities that would not have existed for me had I not become a part of their organization. I can't say enough good things about them. This is a group of very dedicated professionals who care very much for their patients and the well-being of the state of dentistry. Sunrise Dental has helped me at every step of the way on this journey. They are constantly helping me grow, and I'm so appreciative and so fortunate to be associated with them.

My philosophy about dentistry is fairly clear: I treat my patients as if they were family members and/or friends. I use that mindset while making treatment suggestions and plans, whether the suggestion revolves around restoring teeth or restoring smiles. I plan for my patients exactly what I would want to do for my brother or for my children. That's how I go about everything. We always try to keep the patients' best interests in mind. We spend a lot of time offering all of the information that they need, educating them on the situation, and letting them make their own decision regarding the treatment that fits them personally and helps them obtain their goals.

Preparing Your Child for Dental Visits

I'm often asked, "How can I prepare my child for a dental visit?"

Earlier, I mentioned the importance of parenting. Kids respond to certain things based on how they're raised, how they react to adversity, and how they're taught to react to new things. Commonly, I will see a child whose parents have a little anxiety about visiting the dentist. They inadvertently pass down those same anxious feelings to their child. They'll say things like: "If you're good, we'll go get a toy afterwards." The intentions are excellent; however, the child is thinking, "Why do I need to be bribed with this toy, what's going to happen?" The wording might be more productive if it was phrased in a more positive way such as: "Oh, you get to go to the dentist. You're so lucky that you get to go tomorrow." It's something that we have to do and we're going to have fun with it, instead of instilling bad ideas with phrases like "if you are good" or "if you don't cry." If I got told about an upcoming event using this phrase, "If you don't cry when you go here…," I would be fairly skeptical and very hesitant about going. Inadvertently, these anxious feelings get passed on. Children pick up on small things in amazing ways.

The best way to prepare your child for the dentist is to present it not just as a necessary but a fun thing. A trip to the dentist is in the best interest of the child so you might as well make it easy on yourself. You can use phrases like: "The dentist is really nice and a lot of kids have a lot of fun there." Make it exciting for them, and just create that positive energy versus any kind of nervous energy.

In many pediatric dental offices, the parents are not allowed to go to the back with the children because they don't want any inadvertent statements made to the child that might make him or her more anxious. The best way for a parent to act is like it's just another day. Treat it as a very common place for everyone to go and do their important but routine duties, like you're just going to the grocery store or the bank. I know that there are many kids' books that use good wording and can paint their dental experience in a more positive light. Such an investment can be very helpful. There are a number of ways to prepare your child for the first dental visit, but a bribe of some sort is typically a short-term solution at best.

My Child Refuses to Brush…

I've observed that many parents have a similar struggle, along with their children, with getting into the habit of good dental hygiene. It's not at all uncommon for children to want to avoid brushing. It is, however, possible to do a really good brushing using certain dental techniques, such as the "lap to lap and knee to knee technique," which involves the child laying on the laps of two adults, so the teeth can be cleaned easier. However, I always like to tell the parent that a child doesn't want to do anything that's remotely uncomfortable or something that doesn't include instantaneous rewards. Children can feel restrained or helpless letting someone brush their teeth so don't let a child's lack of cooperation deter your intentions. It is in their best interest to have their teeth cleaned.

Children are surrounded by many things that are designed to capture their attention, nearly all of which they would rather do than become good at dental hygiene. As a very conscientious parent, and as an even more conscientious dentist, it's one of those requirements for life that cannot be avoided. As a parent, you need to know that your child doesn't know the world any other way than the way that you teach them. If you instill in them the understanding that taking care of teeth is just a part of life and that they have no alternative—they must brush in order to stay healthy—then that's the attitude they will adopt. And they will know no other way of life.

That thinking also applies to just about anything in life. If a parent instills any value on a consistent basis then the child will adopt it. For instance, if a parent really instills persistence in a kid and the he identifies with it, then when adversity comes along, the child will do his best to persist because he knows no other way. Even though it's a much smaller attribute than determination or anything like that, the same concept applies with brushing the teeth. If a parent makes regular brushing a priority for the child, the child will then make it a personal priority. As the child gets older, he will be used to that habit and won't put it so low on the priority pole.

Parenting is tough work. Children are a major responsibility, but they are also your biggest reward. I take my fatherhood very seriously; I am constantly trying to do what's best for my children and thinking in terms of the big picture. For instance, it's possible that letting them do something other than what they should be doing will keep them happy for the moment, but it only really postpones the problem. There's a saying—if you're too easy on your child when they're young, it makes it harder for them later on in life. If you are more disciplined with them during their early years, the rest of their life tends to be easier. I really think that statement is pretty accurate.

You don't need to deliberately make things hard on your child—life has a way of doing that all by itself. As a parent, you try to give them tools to cope with difficult things, including something that seems to be as miniscule as brushing their teeth. This is the major concept surrounding oral hygiene: if you put in the time with your kids to teach them well, it will pay off later for you and for them.

Baby Teeth

Primary teeth, or baby teeth, for the most part will fall out at some point. For this reason, many people ignore the baby teeth and allow them to become damaged by decay. However, people fail to realize the importance of those little teeth to the child's overall dental health. If a child has a cavity in his early years and the cavity becomes too large, it can cause an infection, and can even make your child become ill. There are actual cases of young children and infants dying from an infection stemming from dental cavities, and nobody wants that.

It could also result in the child having difficulty sleeping and may have to miss school to get the problem addressed. As parents, we don't want our kids to have to suffer through all of these things. Even though the baby teeth will fall out, that doesn't mean that we can neglect them, and it doesn't mean that they're not important.

One of my pediatric patients came into the office and told me that he doesn't smile because he has a big cavity in the front of his teeth. That really struck me. At such a young age, when his identity is just being formed and his self-esteem is taking shape, these important developmental factors are affecting him, and will impact the rest of his life. If the child didn't get this cavity addressed, he would smile less, he would cover his mouth when he laughed, and then start a habit of hiding his mouth. Yes, that tooth will eventually fall out; however, it's an embarrassment to him right now, and he's not living the life that he should be living because of the cavity. It's something that he has to be concerned about every day. On top of that, he's at a higher risk for infection. Once the infection starts, antibiotics may need to be prescribed. Then, down the road, maybe he will need another set of antibiotics for another illness. That set of antibiotics probably won't be as effective, because he already ran a course of it as an adolescent.

These things are part of helping a child grow and develop so that he can live a long, healthy, and happy life. As dentists, we want to get his teeth fixed—we want his teeth to be healthy. Baby teeth are also extremely important as spacers for the adult teeth that come later. If a baby tooth gets a cavity to the point that it must be removed, then the permanent tooth will not grow into the right position. Then the wrongly spaced big tooth will create crowding or spacing issues, which will lead to further negative emotions and self-esteem issues for the child.

Remember, your child might not have the language to express how he feels or the fact that he feels diminished. He probably won't tell you that he's learning bad habits which will follow him throughout all of his adult life. So, as a parent, you've got a duty to do your best for him. Taking care of your child's baby teeth is extremely important in that regard.

YOUR CHILD'S DIET AND HIS DENTAL HEALTH

Just yesterday, a child asked me, "I don't eat a lot of candy, so how do I get cavities?" The cavities are caused by a number of things involving sugars, but the word sugar is understood differently depending on the audience. When you're talking to kids, they're thinking about "sugar" as candy; when you're talking to a biochemist, sugar is a whole different item. Basically, any carbohydrate can cause a cavity—an excess of fast food can cause a lot of cavities. Sticky carbohydrates like chips and Cheetos, and obviously candies such as Jolly Ranchers, can really produce ill effects on your teeth.

Many parents don't understand that every time food is consumed, the pH level in the mouth changes to a level that's more conducive to cavity formation. So, if a child walks around with a bag of chips and nibbles one chip every three minutes for the next four hours, that child will be at a much, much higher risk than the child that sits down and consumes that same volume of chips in a shorter period of time. During the time period when food gets eaten, the pH level changes and promotes cavity formation. So if a child is snacking throughout the day, then their teeth are bathing in a pH level conducive to cavity formation. Also, parents take a big risk by letting their kids walk around with sippy cups and bottles, especially if they're filled with juice or milk. An even worse risk is letting the kids go to sleep without brushing, so those carbohydrates and sugars stay on the teeth all night. The carbohydrates in the juices and milk, sit on the teeth and will lead to more cavities. If we can do some things to protect the child, such as cleaning the teeth or limiting the frequency of the snacking, it can pay big dividends down the road for the child.

Overcoming the Negative Dental Experience

Quite a few patients might attribute a negative dental experience to a particular dentist or blame a dental staff member, but many factors can create a bad experience. The relationship between the dentist and the patient can greatly influence the incident. Of course, there are other contributing factors that often get overlooked. Namely, genetics is a significant influencer that gets forgotten. Your personal genetics can set you up for a bad dental experience if you inherited a low pain threshold or generally sensitive teeth.

Again, your upbringing might be another factor. As I mentioned earlier, if you grew up with poor habits related to oral health (not doing what you were supposed to be doing), or if you heard horror stories from parents or siblings about a bad dental experience, you would probably visit the dental office and expect the visit to be miserable. When you come in tense and afraid, it's difficult to change your expectations. Much of the memory of bad experiences comes from how you generally hold your bad experiences.

Memories of previous experiences can also impact your relationship with a dentist. Maybe there was some pain. Perhaps that dentist wasn't watching your body language and didn't notice that you were experiencing some discomfort. These negative experiences can be cut out of the equation if the right relationship is built between the dentist and the patient. When a dentist is able to create and nurture the trust factor with patients, he can make it all much better and far less traumatic.

Much of that can be addressed early on. Consider, for instance, any individual with red hair, or more particularly individuals with parents or grandparents with red hair. The allele for red hair, if passed down, can express itself in a number of ways. It can give the patient dental anxiety, a greater likelihood of developing cavities along the gum line, and increased tooth sensitivity as well as making them more vulnerable to any sort of addiction. If you can identify these problems early on and explain them to the patient, they will feel as if they are still in control. When you acknowledge their fears as “real” and don’t make them feel foolish, it really helps.

Also, by giving them the necessary information and discussing the things that they might encounter, you can cut out a lot of ill feelings right away. This kind of conversation also allows you to comfort the patient during times when they tend to be more anxious. If they were brought up in a certain way or there were some dramatic events in their life that left them fearful, there are ways to make them feel better about the whole situation.

It’s particularly useful if you can help them realize that both the dentist and the patient want the same end result. Everybody wants to have a good feeling. The goal is generally the same between the dentist and the patient, so once that trust factor is in place, then both sides can work together towards that positive goal. After that, you just keep piling up the positive experiences. Once that first positive experience occurs, and then it happens repeatedly, the bad experience eventually slides down the patient's priority list and even lower on the worry frequency list. A trip to the dentist's office can be a lot more comfortable and a much better experience when the element of trust is introduced and nurtured.

THE VALUE OF A GREAT SMILE

A great smile can change how people feel toward you, but more importantly, it can change the way you feel about yourself. With an improved smile, you feel more confident. Confidence can lead to a number of other positive things. It helps you to appear smarter, more successful, more honest, and even friendlier. When you improve your smile, you are no longer hesitant to smile; you no longer try to hide your smile or teeth behind your hands or a big, bushy mustache. Even though it's a small physical gesture, those smile-hiding behaviors play a huge role in other people's perceptions. If somebody sees you holding back a smile, they could easily mistake that you trying to hide something. Or they could be more inclined to think that you're hiding something or you're not as happy as you really are. Those are major factors, not just in the world of business, but also in the world of personal relationships. Your smile is your introduction to the world.

If you can smile freely and more naturally, it also makes you feel happier inside. I read a lot of literature on mind power, will power, and self-improvement. These books make a big point of saying that if you're smiling and using positive energy, then you're going to end up with more positive results than if you had not used these tools. If you're naturally smiling, then you will feel that same natural happiness in and around you, as will the other people that you encounter. Just try smiling when you're feeling down and you will see what I am referring to. The power of the smile is vastly underrated.

People's lives can be changed instantly by fixing a few teeth here and there. One of the beauties of being a dentist is the ability to change the course of a person's life in an instant, by giving a patient a better smile and helping them to become more self-confident. The patient no longer has to worry about his smile or be self-conscious. In the middle of a conversation, they're not thinking about hiding a certain tooth or hiding their teeth in general. They're in the moment, they're in the conversation, and they can appear more likeable, more personable, and more attentive. It will also be a more enjoyable engagement for them as well. They're no longer worrying about the other person seeing their teeth and wondering if that other person is judging them as a person based on the condition of their teeth.

Tooth repair is a very powerful thing, and it can really influence so many factors in life. One big thing is a job promotion or career success. Often, the more confident person gets promoted. Sometimes, there's a more personal aspect as well, such as the more confident person also getting the girlfriend. Regardless of the situation, that confidence goes such a long way. Until you actually experience it for yourself, you honestly don't know what you're missing. For me as a dentist, it's a great thing to see people's lives change for the better by simply changing their teeth.

By seeing the life experiences that I'm able to improve, I get to experience a great deal of excitement and pride in doing what I do. Sure, dentists are able to fix a cavity or remove a tooth, but out of the many things that a dentist can do, the most fun part of my job includes changing people's life circumstances and even altering their entire life path. It's an exciting thing to be able to say that we, as an office, can turn somebody's life around—and also the lives of their spouse and children—that we can apply our knowledge and training to make life better for people. It's so rewarding.

Signs of Tooth Erosion

Tooth erosion can sneak up on you if you don't watch for it. There are numerous signs of tooth erosion, but the bigger concern is the underlying reason for that erosion, whether it's grinding (bruxism) or the effect of acidic beverages, etc. One of my major concerns when I examine patients is any sign of acid reflux disease (GERD). A dentist should be able to identify this condition with relative ease.

GERD has a serious impact on your teeth as well as your whole digestive system, which is why it should be identified as soon as possible. If your body is in constant acid reflux mode, regular processes become much more difficult. Things like digesting food and basic bodily comfort become a lot tougher; GERD detracts from your life. If acid is eroding your teeth, imagine what it could be doing to the soft tissues of your esophagus.

When dentists see these signs in patients, we can suggest the practice of keeping a dietary journal to help identify one of the numerous causes or triggers of the reflux: spicy food, greasy food, alcohol, eating just before bedtime, etc. Once we identify the triggers, then we can reduce or moderate those items in the diet to create a more pleasurable life for the individual.

All of these related factors of acid reflux are worth discussing with patients at length. We can help them identify the cause of the condition and then move forward. Patients should remember that big systemic issues identified by your dentist can really, really impact your overall health. With the right counseling, we can limit the effects of issues such as tooth erosion, which is sometimes caused by the effects of acidic beverages. For instance, you might think that after you drink orange juice, you should brush your teeth. However, due to the chemistry in your mouth (more acidity plus saliva changes the pH of the mouth), it's best to not brush your teeth for 30 minutes after drinking orange juice. A simple talk with your dentist about this issue can go a long way toward preventing a lot of future negative effects before they happen. As a dentist, I feel like one of my main goals is to get the dentition to a place where people can eat what they want to eat without thinking about their teeth.

Missing Teeth

Many people don't understand the importance of individual teeth to your health. For example, if you're missing a rear molar, there are consequences. When you lose one tooth, the other teeth begin to shift and move to compensate for the missing tooth. This causes you to lose chewing power, possibly develop jaw soreness, cause other teeth to move and make them more susceptible to root sensitivity, or not to mention looking completely different with no tooth. So, what do you do? Well, there are several available options.

1. We could recommend a retainer or a partial denture, which is the least expensive option.
2. We might suggest a bridge, so adjacent teeth are crowned and a tooth is placed in the space between those two.
3. I often suggest or recommend an implant because of their current success rates. Recently, implants have really improved and become popular. They are highly successful, highly durable, and provide amazing longevity

and results. However, there's also the cost factor to be considered, which can be a game-changer for many.

Many factors come into play when a patient is choosing restoration options for missing teeth, especially regarding the anterior (visible) teeth; the effects on these teeth focus less on chewing power and more on aesthetics. Change in somebody's anterior smile or front teeth, can have a number of ill effects, namely on the way that a patient regards himself and the way that others perceive him. Others may misconstrue a missing tooth in the front with a number of bad things. While I don't know precisely what people think, assumptions are often made when somebody has a missing front tooth.

Some patients don't even know that they have options. If they can just understand those options, they can start taking steps to making their life better. Some patients don't find any change in the way they see themselves so they don't want any treatment. As long as the patients know their options, they are the ones who always make the ultimate decision.

For example, if the problem is a financial obstacle, then they can start saving for it. Just getting some missing teeth replaced can boost an individual's confidence in a major, major way. Something as simple as fixing a broken tooth can help steer their life in a more optimistic direction. Once they can get that tooth restored, they will feel more confident, and then the sky's the limit. They can get a better job and feel happier in general, but the process starts with exploring the available options. I know I'm beating a dead horse here but it can't be said enough how big this can be.

Dental Work and Its Longevity

I hear this question quite often in reference to recent dental work: "How long will it last?" In all honesty, the answer is really unknown to the dentist. In simple procedures like fillings, the success can be predicted relatively well. If it's something like a crown from a tooth that's had a big cavity, a precise answer to those questions is a little bit more difficult. Generally, fillings and crown procedures are done with the intention and attempt to make them last a lifetime. I occasionally give a very cynical response to the length of time that dental restorations and repairs will last, like "as long as you let it."

Dentists can fix just about anything. For most issues that we fix, if nothing was eaten ever again, that crown would generally last forever; but in reality, not eating anything is not what we are looking for here. Remember, your teeth are tools, and hopefully, they are also jewels that sparkle and shine. There is no ideal way to predict the longevity of a restoration, because it depends on how the teeth are used and/or abused or what the patient eats.

Nor do we know everything that the patient does. Maybe they have a habit like biting their fingernails that would chip a front filling; maybe they have a habit of chewing on hardened pizza crusts or chewing on ice (this is a big one). Regarding fillings, I can say with confidence that they will last a very, very long time. Most dentists offer some sort of guarantee on fillings and crowns. However, some cases are a lot more difficult for predicting the longevity, based on a lack of knowledge about the dietary environment that's occurring or the dietary attack on the teeth.

Dentists can give recommendations and let patients know what will be harmful. However, if the patient chews ice every single day, that habit makes it difficult to predict the length of time that a restoration will last under the attack of the ice. As a dentist, all I can do is give the best recommendation that I see. Remember this: your own natural teeth were meant to last for an entire lifetime.

Dental Cleanings

Every patient is different in terms of the timing of their dental cleaning. This frequency of cleanings would be determined by the dentist. However, I think the general population sometimes underrates the importance of clean teeth. People think, "Oh, I haven't had a cavity in x number of years, so I don't really need to go to the dentist." Without knowing it, those people are probably dealing with tartar build-up, also known as calculus—not to be confused with the math subject. Dental calculus builds up on teeth and becomes hard like concrete. It builds up underneath the gums, particularly on the back side of the front bottom teeth, and people don't think much about it until there's an underlying problem to fix. What's really happening is that your body is trying to fight that foreign debris; but in doing so, it is basically killing off some of the bone around the teeth. So the teeth then lose support.

I like to explain the concept with this illustration: it's like setting up an umbrella in the sand at the beach. If you bury that umbrella's pole into only a foot of sand, then that umbrella will be pretty unstable. Burying that pole into a few feet of sand makes the umbrella much more stable. The same thing is true about your teeth. As you lose bone around your teeth, the stability of your teeth starts to decline. When that begins to happen, your teeth become unstable and loose pretty quickly, and there's not much for a dentist to do to get the bone back. Our hands are tied as far as treatment options. Our best defense in this case is prevention.

People often think that they can just go in and get the problem fixed, but with bone loss, it's very difficult to fix the problem to a point where it's restored "like new." Here it is in a nutshell: dental cleanings prevent bone loss. The idea is to keep debris off your teeth so that your body is not trying to fight that foreign substance; then you won't experience bone loss, or you won't get any inflammation.

Inflammation and bone loss from periodontal disease or gum disease can create worse problems throughout your body. Gum disease has been shown to contribute to a higher risk of certain illnesses and medical issues: stroke, heart attack, heart disease, etc. So, take an hour every few months and go get your teeth cleaned, and avoid bone loss. The higher risk of stroke and heart attack is also something not to take lightly either. That's what makes a dental cleaning one of the more important priorities for you in the course of a day.

Cleaning Beyond the Teeth and Gums

I'd like to speak briefly about the subject of bad breath, which is a huge problem in society. The worst part is that the people who suffer from bad breath are often the most unaware of it. A number of simple things can be done to alleviate bad breath.

Keep your teeth squeaky clean: Make sure to regularly clean and floss your teeth. Don't postpone making appointments for your dental checkups if you want to keep your teeth healthy. Rotting food between your teeth can't smell pretty.

Deal with cavities: The smell of a deep cavity is not desirable for anybody, so obviously it's necessary to get your cavities addressed, along with all of the unhealthy things in your mouth.

It's a big and important job to keep your teeth clean, keep your gums healthy, and then floss your teeth. Any plaque that's left in between your teeth will resonate for as long as it's left there. If you think about food that's left unattended for a few days, the residual scenario is usually not the best.

Brush your tongue: A lot of bacteria and debris can get embedded in your tongue, so make sure to brush it. Basically, sticking out your tongue and giving it a little scrub will be extremely helpful.

Use mouthwash for temporary odors: Beyond the odor of decaying debris, there's also the odor that comes from your diet. If you eat a lot of garlic and onions, those things will cause temporary bad breath, but they can be alleviated with a mouthwash or green tea, or by eating something else that replaces the scent (mint leaves).

Fast food—mouth odor's buddy: Eating a lot of fast food allows a lot of plaque to stick to your teeth, which causes residual bad breath. It also resonates even after digestion similar to when you are dehydrated.

Stay hydrated: If your mouth is very dry and you're dehydrated, you're going to pick up some chemicals that don't give off the best odor.

All of these important things are relatively easy to do and can be done fairly quickly. Taking these steps can help you change how you feel and how you talk to people.

FINALLY... A FEW LAST WORDS

Because I love my profession, I'm very much interested in the direction and focus of dentistry in the future. I believe that dentistry will become very family-oriented and personable, as more and more dentists open their own offices and get out into the working field. I think there will be a higher value placed on the personable dentist, who will work to create a positive relationship and view the patient as a whole, rather than just as a set of teeth.

Actually, that's how I see dentistry fitting into healthcare as a whole. Your mouth is such a major part of everything we do as human beings — it's the gateway to our bodies. It stands to reason, and scientific research has shown, that the condition of your mouth (your oral health) has a major influence on your overall physical health as well as your overall emotional well-being and self-confidence. In the future, I'm hopeful that the role of dentistry fits within healthcare as just one piece of a bigger picture.

(This content should be used for informational purposes only. It does not create a doctor-patient relationship with any reader and should not be construed as medical advice. If you need medical advice, please contact a doctor in your community who can assess the specifics of your situation.)

9

Honesty And Quality In Dental Care And Giving Back To The Community

by Roya N. Akbar, D.M.D.

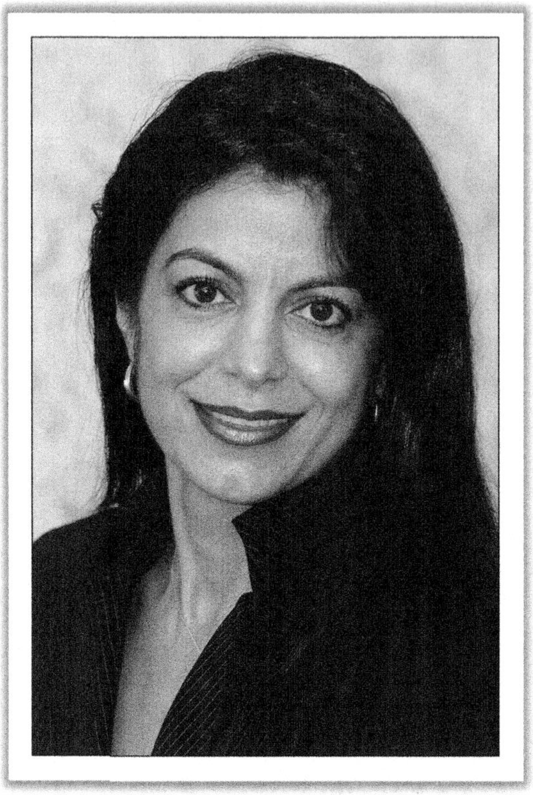

Roya N. Akbar, D.M.D.
R.A. Dental Studio
Marietta, Georgia
www.drakbar.com

Dr. Roya Akbar is considered to be among the top dentists in the greater Atlanta, GA area. Her specialized training – combined with the latest technology and techniques – provides her patients with compassionate care and professional expertise.

After graduating with a bachelor's degree of Science and Biology from Brenau University in Gainesville, Georgia, she went on to attend the Medical College of Georgia in Augusta, where she received her D.M.D. From there, Dr. Akbar furthered her studies at Oklahoma University in Oklahoma City, where she received a postgraduate degree in advanced education in general dentistry. She was licensed by the Georgia Board of Dentistry in 1990, and begin practicing in Atlanta by 1991.

She is also licensed through D.O.C.S. to perform oral conscious sedation, allowing her to offer quality care to many patients who may otherwise go untreated due to anxiety or time restraints. Her professional memberships include: the American Dental Association, the Georgia Dental Association, the American Academy of Cosmetic Dentistry, the Seattle Study Club of Atlanta and the Dental Organization of Conscious Sedation.

An avid runner, Dr. Roya Akbar takes time almost every day to run, and also ran the New York Marathon in 2008. She also participates in multiple free dental days throughout the year. During the free dental days, 200 to 300 patients are seen in a day. Her philanthropic work with the Green Foundation has earned her a mention in Time Magazine.

Helping others is something that Dr. Roya Akbar takes very seriously. The wish of a dying young girl was that she could have a beautiful smile for all to see. She knew it was close to the end, and her wish was granted by Dr. Akbar. Just months before the girl passed away, she gave that young girl a beautiful smile.

Honesty And Quality In Dental Care And Giving Back To The Community

Coming To The United States Enabled Me To Follow My Dreams And Aspirations

I was born in Iran and had a very happy childhood as the middle child in a close-knit family of five. I began high school in Iran before arriving in the United States at the age of 14, where I finished high school. When my family came to the United States, the plan was not for us to stay here. We were planning to receive an education, and then return to the place where I was born. As life would have it, we were thrown a curve ball. There was a revolution in Iran and as a result of all the political changes taking place, all funds were cut off to thousands of Iranian students.

I found myself in a position where I didn't have any type of financial support, and I decided, as did so many other Iranian students, that failure was not an option. After all, this is the way we were brought up. All I did was study, because Iranian students like myself had no other choice but to survive and be the best students. As a result, today the Iranian American community is one of the most successful immigrant communities in America. We had no choice but to succeed.

When I came to the United States, my family believed it was a country full of opportunity. My parents wanted all of their children to do well in life, and receiving an education was very important to us. Even though everyone goes through struggles in life, my parents taught us that you do what you must to excel and to reach your goals.

Due to the fact that I was so focused on my education and doing well in school, I didn't have much of a social life. I didn't participate in many social activities in high school, nor did I attend my Prom. Instead, I spent most of my time in the Chemistry lab. Because I didn't have a social life, I could be more focused, which eventually led to the success I have today.

After high school, I attended Brenau University as an undergraduate. I graduated from college when I was 19 years old. I went to the Medical College of Georgia to study to become a physician's assistant (PA), but my heart was always set on going to dental school.

I applied to dental school several times before I was accepted to the dental program at the Medical College of Georgia. I often thought that the reason for getting rejected was that I was viewed as too young and not mature enough for the grueling course load. After I graduated, I completed a one-year residency in general dentistry in Oklahoma City before returning to Georgia.

Despite the aforementioned curve ball, coming to the United States was the event that had the greatest influence on my life. I learned how to adapt to a new country and it enabled me to follow my dreams and aspirations. I believed that I could be whoever I wanted to be, and do well in life as long as I worked hard for it.

As long as I can remember, I have always wanted to be a dentist and it must have been in my genes. I have memories from when I was eight or nine years old, when I would pretend to be a physician or a dentist. I had a little white coat and everything that goes along with it. With the neighborhood kids, I would examine them and prescribe medication. Sometimes, I would even pretend that I was performing surgery or extracting a tooth using my dad's pliers (I actually did pull a baby tooth once but the rest was just make believe).

It must be the same for my youngest daughter because she wants to become an Orthodontist. I tell her, "To become a dentist, you must be a very patient person, be able to work with your hands, and be very articulate." I have also explained to her that I have found dentistry to be very fulfilling. When I am able to improve a person's smile, I feel as if I have accomplished something powerful, and they have been given another chance to further enhance their quality of life. You really can change a person's life through dentistry.

I've been married to my wonderful husband Paul for nearly 25 years, and we have three children: Kameron, Lily, and Jasmine. Two of our children attend college and the youngest just entered high school. Kameron is starting his third year at Georgia Tech, and Lily started the second year as an honor student at Georgia State. Jasmine begins high school this upcoming year.

My Philosophy of Dentistry and Patient Care

As a dentist, when a patient walks through your doors, you must be very honest and truthful about the treatment that you can offer them. Trust is the most important part of dentistry. A patient must trust you for you to be able to treat him or her. You could be an incredible dentist, but if the patient doesn't trust you, it's worthless.

Also, as a comprehensive dentist, I'm not a one-trick pony. I think your mouth is the gateway to your body. Mouth and body connection is very important because everything connects together; people don't often realize that if their mouth is not healthy, they will not be healthy people. Oral health relates to a number of health conditions such as diabetes, heart disease, endocarditis, and pregnancy. For example, if a person has a lot of build-up on their teeth and their gums subsequently become infected, then disease can spread to other areas of the body and cause serious health issues. After infection sets in, gum disease and heart disease go hand-in-hand. If a patient has diabetes as well as periodontal disease, these issues will surely cause bone loss.

In comprehensive dentistry, you tell patients exactly what they need to have done and how much it will cost. To me, comprehensive dentistry is extremely important for providing patients with the best care, which is the priority. Also, patient education is a very important element for providing a positive office experience and personalized dental care. I believe a dentist needs to tell the patient about the work that's necessary rather than what the patient may want to hear, because the patient is often unable to see the entire picture. I always tell new patients what I believe needs to be done, and all too often the patient will say, "My old dentist didn't tell me this."

My philosophy is never to judge a patient by the clothes they wear or the way they speak, to always provide the patient with the best care, regardless of the price. Tell the patient about the treatment that is best for that patient, and let the patient decide how to proceed. I'll say, "This treatment (x) is the best thing for you. You could get by with this option (y), but this (x) is the ultimate way that I would go because, if you settled for (y), you would waste a lot of money and perhaps lose a tooth. At times, it might be more beneficial to extract a tooth and place an implant, rather than have a large filling done which might need a root canal later, and face the possibility of the tooth failing in the future." Lack of honesty with a patient could mean that they would pay a lot more for additional treatments, only to be unhappy in the end. Painting the full picture for the patient, regardless of the price, is always the best way to practice dentistry. My philosophy has paid off in that I have very loyal patients and many consider me a friend.

Although I'm a general practitioner, I love dental surgery. I'm constantly in study clubs and discussions with friends about the gore of dentistry – jumping in, sweating it out, working through the fear. As a result, some of my colleagues send me their difficult cases. I perform a great number of full mouth reconstructions and difficult surgeries that most general dentists avoid. I always refer the patients back to their original dentists, which is great for me, because those dentists have placed their trust in me and as a result they continue to send patients to me. They don't want to lose their patients by sending them to a dentist who will try to keep the patient in his or her own practice.

ENVISIONING THE FUTURE OF DENTISTRY

The future of dentistry lies in one word: digital. From impressions to scanners to x-rays, you name the procedure, and it is digital. Digital impressions make dentistry a lot easier. I'm hoping for a soundless drill because that would be awesome. The sound of drilling is one of the chief complaints from many patients. There is also a saliva test in process, to determine who's at risk for certain diseases or disorders. It's not fully workable, but it is close. I think there's another procedure in development that would permit us to grow a real tooth for replacement, rather than installing another titanium implant. It would be more like a natural tooth. Another advancement needing improvement is protection from tooth decay for babies, even before they begin to cut their primary teeth.

The business side of dentistry is also changing in a big way. Group-managed practices are popping up on every corner, like Walmart's of the dental industry. Many older dentists are finding it more difficult to remain in practice when they must compete with these group-managed practices, in addition to the changing insurance rules with the new Affordable Care Act. Many patients are price shopping, but people are not receiving the higher level of dental care provided by the private practitioner. Having interviewed dentists who work in these group-managed practices, I've heard repeatedly from these dentists that they must meet production quota by placing a crown on a tooth, when they feel the best course of action for the patient would be a filling. Since the crown pays more, the crown is done.

I don't know if patients are being short-changed with this type of dental care. Unfortunately, that is the direction taken by dentistry in the last few years. It will likely continue in that direction for a number of years before we have a backlash, and people will begin to once again appreciate the quality of care provided by a general practitioner. Dentists like myself are already established and have a very large pool of patients. For the new dentists entering the field, I think the market has drastically changed for them. That is an unfortunate aspect of the business side of dentistry.

Comfort (or Sedation) Dentistry

Three factors commonly stop people from going to the dentist: fear, time, and money. In sedation dentistry, we use medication to help the patient relax during the dental procedure. It's very simple. We also take additional steps to make the patient more comfortable, such as providing blankets, headphones, and music. When patients are comfortable, the dentist's life is also made a lot easier and the procedure goes a lot faster. Everything takes less time.

There are several types of sedation available in dentistry, depending on the patient's need. First, laughing gas is sufficient for most patients. For patients who are a little more anxious, a second type of sedation (conscious sedation) is available. This type of sedation is when the patient is given oral medication to help them relax. They are responsive and conscious but relaxed; they do not remember very much, if anything, about the procedure. Often times, the patient will be so relaxed that they fall asleep. During deep sedation, the third option, an IV is used to sedate the patient.

In my own practice, I use conscious sedation - I love it and my patients love it as well. Many times, I perform the procedure, call to check on the patient, and the patient does not remember the visit to the office at all. The medicine has an amnesia effect, so the patient does not even recall having the procedure. It can also help patients who have a severe gag reflex. If the patient has a difficult time getting numb, you use a lot less anesthetic when using oral medication to help them relax. Another benefit is that the patient does not hear or remember the sound of the drill, which is a problem for many patients. If someone has had a bad experience in the past, sedation helps that patient deal with their fears so they can get the necessary dental treatments to obtain a healthy mouth.

Because of the oral sedation that I can offer my patients, we are able to perform several treatments in one visit. For example, whenever I do sedation dentistry, I may only schedule two patients for the day – one patient in the morning, and one patient in the afternoon. In the morning, I start at about 6:30 a.m. getting the patient comfortable. I'll be finished with the morning patient by 11:30 a.m. The afternoon patient starts at 12:30 p.m.

Cosmetic Dentistry and Smile Improvement

Cosmetic dentistry focuses on the appearance of the teeth and the enhancement of a person's smile. Since it's not a dentistry specialty, a dentist who focuses in this area can't officially say, "I'm a cosmetic dentist." Everybody's a cosmetic dentist if you say that, but it does take many, many years of extensive training and experience to perform excellent cosmetic dental procedures; otherwise, it could be a disaster. When it comes to cosmetic dentistry, the dentist is like the conductor of an orchestra. You must be able to communicate with the patient and your lab technician, and above all, you need to have an eye for the work.

A dentist must listen to the patient to discover what he or she wants. If the patient says, "I would like this procedure because I want to look this way," you must be able to listen and understand. Many people want to have ceramic white teeth but to me, that's unnatural. So although it's always about fulfilling a patient's needs, it's my responsibility to educate and inform the patient of the possible ramifications of their decision. Listening to the patient's requests and properly understanding their needs are crucial in achieving a successful outcome.

With cosmetic dentistry, depending on the procedure, you can have subtle or drastic changes in the appearance of the smile, and the results can be surprising. In-Office teeth whitening is a very simple cosmetic procedure. It enhances your beauty, your smile, and gives one a youthful appearance better than any cosmetic procedure can do. Other procedures include composite bonding, porcelain or composite veneers, simple tooth re-shaping, or tooth re-contouring.

Some procedures are simple and can be done in one visit, but they make such a big difference in someone's life. For example, cosmetic gum re-contouring is a procedure that corrects a very gummy smile. The dentist uses a laser to gently remove excessive gum tissue and sculpt a more harmonious, attractive smile. That makes a huge difference in someone's smile. You can also insert porcelain bridges to replace missing teeth or use dental implants. Improving a person's smile can have a substantial effect on their life and confidence.

Old and Discolored Fillings

Let's assume that you have a few old silver fillings and you want to replace them with something more aesthetically pleasing. Dentists can replace these silver fillings with tooth-colored fillings. If you have a very large filling, the best choice would be to conserve the tooth structure by using a porcelain onlay or inlay rather than a full-coverage crown. Many dentists place crowns because they may not feel comfortable using the techniques involved in doing porcelain onlays and inlays. Veneers are more technique-sensitive and more time-consuming than crowns, because the cuts have to be done a certain way.

I personally prefer doing onlays and inlays as opposed to doing a crown, because they truly help the patient preserve the tooth structure. When you do a crown, you must do more tooth reduction versus inlays and onlays. When you do tooth reduction, you cause patients to have more sensitivity. If you can do inlays and onlays, they're really the best way to get rid of unattractive and discolored fillings.

Porcelain Veneers and Smile Improvement

Stated very simply, a porcelain veneer is a thin shell of porcelain that covers and is bonded to the tooth. A veneer changes the color, the shape, and the alignment of your tooth. It truly changes the appearance of your smile. If you have any chipped areas, it restores the chipped or uneven teeth. If you have a noticeable space in between your teeth, you can close that space with veneers. If your teeth are worn down, veneers can restore the worn areas to make a huge difference in your smile.

Everything connects together with the power of a great and beautiful smile. The first thing that people notice about you is your smile, especially your teeth. People remember you from your smile and it has a huge impact on your success in both your personal and your business relationships. If you have crooked teeth or discolored teeth, then that is what people will notice about you. An attractive smile makes a big difference, gives you more confidence, and helps you to become more noticed by people, but in a positive way.

I helped one handsome young man when he was 15 years of age. He had fluorosis (brownish discoloration from overexposure to fluoride) on all his teeth and his mother couldn't afford expensive dental procedures. I did something much simpler and as effective for him. Rather than porcelain veneers, I applied composite bonding. The result was stunning and that changed him in such positive way. Now, he has a really big smile; he's more confident and happy in life and very glad to be on the football team.

One of my other patients was a beautiful 81-year-old woman whose last dental visit was 30 years prior. She came to the office and said, "I've been through a lot in my life and I hate my smile."She had discolored teeth with many cavities and dental issues. We started by making her gums healthy which provide the foundation for a healthy mouth. We then took care of her cavities and then she said, "Doc, I want to look good - I want to do something with my front teeth. Money is not important. Just make me look good and give me the best smile possible." I went through the different options with her. We reconstructed her whole smile and you should see her now; after it was done, she said, "Just put me on your wall as a poster child." She's a different woman now; she's healthy, and very happy, and smiles often. When she comes to the office, she brings a lot of joy and love and positive energy with her.

To me, it doesn't matter how old you are, because beauty is beauty. Your first impression is important, and it is a lasting impression. People will remember you. That is my philosophy for having a pretty smile.

GUM DISEASE

"What is gum disease? What is gingivitis? How do we get it? How can I prevent it?" "How is it treated?" We hear these questions quite often in the dental office.

Gingivitis means "inflammation of the gums". When plaque and bacteria are not thoroughly removed from the teeth, the tissue can respond by becoming red, swollen and inflamed, resulting in gingivitis. Gingivitis is easily treatable with proper brushing and flossing. However, if ignored, the plaque continues to accumulate on the teeth and eventually results in the formation of tartar, which is a very hard substance full of bacteria and toxins. Once tartar forms on the teeth, it is not easily removed with brushing and flossing alone; it must be removed with professional dental cleanings. If it is not removed, the tartar continues to adhere to the teeth, causing the gums to become more swollen and to bleed. Bleeding gums are a sign of periodontal (gum) disease and infection. If the infection is left untreated, it will eventually result in bone loss around the teeth, which can then lead to eventual tooth loss. Studies now also show that there is a direct oral-systemic link between gum disease and other diseases. People with gum disease have a greater chance of having heart disease, stroke, high blood pressure and uncontrolled diabetes.

There are different stages of gum disease: early, moderate, and advanced. If gum disease is treated in the early stage, you can prevent further bone loss from occurring around the teeth. If ignored, the teeth will become loose and mobile, eventually resulting in tooth loss.

Some people may say, "It's not hurting me. Why do I need treatment?" Gum disease can be silent; some people may not even know they have a problem until their dentist tells them, or until they begin to show signs of bone loss, such as loose or mobile teeth. When you visit your dentist, they should do a thorough exam of your gums each year. This is done by taking dental x-rays that enable them to see the bone that supports the teeth, and also by using a special tiny ruler that is placed under the gum tissue to measure the space between the tooth and the gum; this allows them to determine the bone levels around each tooth. In a healthy mouth, the bone levels should be between 1 to 3 mm and no bleeding should be present. People with gum disease will have measurements greater than 4 mm, which means that a pocket has formed around the tooth and the gums will bleed due to the infection present. The deeper the pocket, the more bone loss has occurred around the tooth. Gum disease is treatable but not curable. This means that the bone loss is permanent, but with proper treatment you can stabilize gum disease and prevent further bone loss from occurring.

If you have been diagnosed with gum disease, depending on the severity, your dentist will likely recommend a form of nonsurgical periodontal therapy, called Scaling and Root Planing. This is a special type of dental cleaning that involves removing all of the tartar and bacteria from under the gums, which can then allow the gum tissue to heal and reattach to the tooth so that the pockets will shrink back to a normal, healthy depth. People with a history of gum disease will need to be very diligent with proper homecare and regular periodontal maintenance cleanings every 3 to 4 months, to make sure the disease continues to be stabilized. By doing so, this will help to ensure that you keep your teeth for many years to come.

Clenching and Tooth Grinding (Bruxism)

Many people are unaware that they might be clenching or grinding their teeth, as it often occurs at night when a person is sleeping. Studies have shown that as many as 90% of the population grind or clench their teeth. People are also more likely to grind their teeth if they are under a lot of pressure or stress. A simple evaluation by your dentist can determine if you might have this habit.

If you clench and grind your teeth, the resulting pressure and forces can damage the tooth structure, resulting in uneven wear, cracks in the teeth, damage to your jaw joints, and even breakage of teeth.

If left untreated, the teeth will continue to lose more and more tooth structure over time. The teeth will continue to wear down, eventually becoming shorter and shorter. You may have seen an older person, or sometimes even a young person, with very short teeth; they are most likely grinding their teeth.

Bruxism, or teeth grinding, can be prevented by simply providing the patient with a special type of appliance called a "bite guard' that is usually worn at night while the patient sleeps. This special guard is custom-fitted to a person's mouth and allows the teeth to be protected, and prevents further damage to the tooth structure.

Treatment Options for Missing Teeth

Replacing missing or unsalvageable teeth involves using implants, bridges and dentures to enhance your appearance and oral health. If you have any missing teeth, it may impact the remainder of your teeth and the way your teeth bite together. Your teeth may shift, creating spaces that food can get trapped in. This can substantially increase your risk of gum disease and tooth decay. Your facial muscles may also become saggy if many of your teeth are missing. This can impact your speech as well as your looks.

The number of teeth missing makes a big difference in the way that we plan your treatment. If you have one missing tooth, you have several options for replacing that tooth, from an implant to a bridge to a partial denture. If the adjacent teeth have never experienced any restorative work, an implant is the ideal solution. Before placing a bridge, we would need to precisely shape the adjacent teeth; however, if we use an implant, we would not need to touch the adjacent teeth. In many cases, once we place the implant, we let the area heal and allow the bone to integrate around the implant. We then fabricate a custom abutment and a crown on top of the implant. That's the best option if you're missing one tooth.

If you're missing numerous teeth or have unsalvageable teeth, there are a number of options available. Dentures are possible, but choosing dentures is not an option that we recommend for all patients. If you have an existing upper and lower denture and are unhappy with them, I would recommend placing implants. You can do what we call implant-supported dentures. We place a few implants and the denture snaps into the implants. This helps the function of the teeth, since the denture doesn't move when you chew or speak. The implants stabilize the denture.

I think that dentures make it very difficult for patients to function, especially as they get older. It especially affects seniors' ability to chew and eat. Let's assume that you come to my office with a partial on the upper and a partial on the lower, but you have few natural teeth and they are not in good condition. I will tell you that you can have a set of dentures (which I do not recommend), or we can remove the unhealthy teeth, place a few implants, and then create implant-supported dentures.

If you are missing many teeth, have no teeth, or have bad gums, Implant Supported Dentures may be a great option for you. I generally recommend placing a minimum of 5 implants in the lower jaw and 6 in the upper jaw to ensure maximum stability and reduce the possibility of a failure. A fixed prosthesis is then attached to a titanium bar which snaps into these implants. With a fixed prosthesis, there are no removable items in your mouth. While it is a good procedure for many patients who don't want something removable, it is also cost-prohibitive for many of them. But in spite of its cost, I still believe in providing the patient with all their options, and let the patient make the decision.

Giving Back to the Community

My passion is performing smile makeovers, and when an opportunity presents itself, offering that service to people who cannot afford the expense of cosmetic dentistry. I believe in giving back to your community, and it's truly satisfying to perform charitable dentistry for people in need. Several weekends every year, I am provided the chance to work with various dentists treating as many as 200 to 300 patients on a weekend through a program known by a number of names – Dentistry from the Heart, Give Back a Smile, and Community of Smiles. We begin early in the morning and provide free dentistry until the last patient is seen, no matter how long it takes. I usually perform surgical extractions for people whose teeth are beyond restoration. People line up the night before to receive these vital services. I was also honored in Time Magazine for my contribution to the Dream Foundation, when I helped a local woman restore her teeth. Her teeth had been ravaged by years of chemotherapy and radiation and I felt privileged to have that opportunity.

At other times, I have helped battered women restore their smiles, giving them back the confidence they had lost. Every dentist and every clinician should give back to the community, and fortunately many step up to this honor.

I do my best to help patients who fall into hardship. During the recession a few years ago, we told a number of patients who were going through financial stress, "Just come in and let's maintain your dental health. There's no charge for you to just maintain the teeth you already have. Whenever you're ready financially, you can get your new smile." We maintain their oral health at no charge until they can financially afford treatment and are back on their feet again. The focus of dentistry should never be only about making money.

Enjoying My Job

I really, really love what I do and enjoy it every day. If I had to do it all over again, I certainly would. There's not a day that goes by when I feel like I "have" to go see this patient or I "must" do this or that. I take it one day at a time, and I have a great time seeing my patients. I enjoy my patients, the amazing team we have working for us, and my dental colleagues. For me, it's never felt like a job. It's fun, because I always enjoy the next challenge and I relish each one. The more difficult the case, the more excited I become when putting a plan together and creating a new smile for my patient, and watching them become more confident. Dentistry should never be viewed as an occupation, it is a career and we should all be so lucky to love what we do.

On the other hand, dentistry is very different from other careers in medicine. Dentists have to work in a very confined area that includes a significant amount of stress. If you don't love dentistry, you will become a miserable person in this profession. If you wish to pursue dentistry as a career, I recommend working in a dental office to see if it is what you want to do for the rest of your life. I think that is the best advice I can give to anyone considering dentistry as a career path.

Dentistry is not all about techniques; you have to have a kind heart. You also have to love the work and the people, be a very caring and loving person, and have a lot of patience.

Being a dentist is wonderful. I am blessed to love what I do each day. Being a dentist is who I am and who I want to be.

(This content should be used for informational purposes only. It does not create a doctor-patient relationship with any reader and should not be construed as medical advice. If you need medical advice, please contact a doctor in your community who can assess the specifics of your situation.)

10

How You Grow Up Doesn't Matter… It's The Dream That Matters

by Elias J. Achey, Jr., D.M.D.

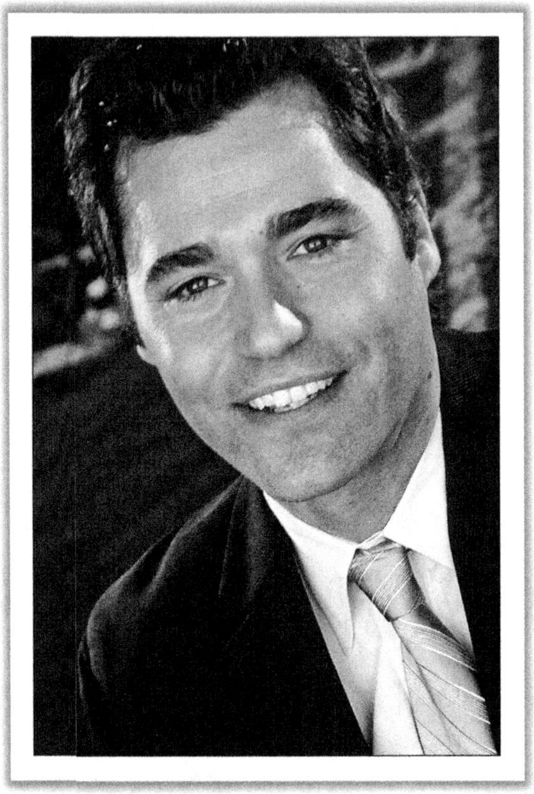

Elias J. Achey, Jr., D.M.D.

Infinity Dental Partners
Spring Lake, Michigan
www. infinitydentalpartners.com

Dr. Elias J. Achey, Jr. graduated from the University of Alabama School of Dentistry at Birmingham in 2006 and moved to West Michigan to practice near extended family. Shortly after his journey north, he married a beautiful Mississippi southern belle, Ann Claire, and they now have two beautiful children, Margot and Elias, Jr.

Unhappy with the traditional model of practice ownership and management, Dr. Achey quickly sought a way to empower team members and live for a larger vision. He discovered Next Level Practice at the inception of his career and, along with Dr. Jared Van Ittersum, experienced explosive growth not only in his practice, but in his personal life. Together, the two set out with the vision that every doctor should experience the bliss they had achieved.

Practicing clinical dentistry while simultaneously managing a large group practice certainly keeps him busy, but he finds great balance with his family at their farmhouse they built in 2014. If he is not with a patient, at a meeting or on a Skype with team members, you can find him on a tractor, out in the woods with his kids, or enjoying the country in his free time.

HOW YOU GROW UP DOESN'T MATTER… IT'S THE DREAM THAT MATTERS

A ROUGH BEGINNING

I grew up in San Bernardino, California, and we were constantly moving. My mom was addicted to drugs, and life was like a roller coaster, up and down. My dad has been a millionaire three times, and he lost it all three times.

One time stands out: when I was in first grade and my dad lost it all. We didn't have a place to live, and we ended up in a shelter that was just like a big warehouse. That was a really weird point in my life, but living through those difficult times now empowers me, and the memories help push me forward to the life I live today.

While in this low-income housing, my dad got his real estate license and started buying and selling property. Things got a little bit better for us, and we were able to move out of there to a better area of California.

While growing up, I had a couple of best friends. We would play baseball in the street, and we had our own BMX bikes and Oakleys when they first came out. We had our own little BMX gang. We'd spend our days outside and jump our bikes all day long, just having a good time.

Unfortunately, that's when my mom started doing drugs. Without her supervision, I stopped going to school because I enjoyed riding bikes more than I enjoyed going to school. I would pretend to go, but instead, I'd get on my bike and take off. Then I'd meet my friends after they got out of school.

It was during that time that I started getting involved with gangs, and I started going down the wrong road. I never did drugs, but I started affiliating with the wrong crowd. It was a blessing in disguise that my dad lost his company and we moved from California to Alabama.

My dad had a client in Alabama who agreed to work with my dad to develop a property that he owned. So at that point, my dad just closed the doors, packed everything up, and we drove to Alabama in an '89 Ford Probe. To this day, I remember the car being packed with all our stuff, as well as me, my mom, and my little dog, Oreo. We went from this booming metropolitan area of San Bernardino to a town with two traffic lights in Alabama.

Moving to Alabama and Becoming a Dentist Saved My Life

I feel that move helped me to become a man and not behave like a kid. I started learning manners, and I started learning about life. I went back to school, and I had to get tutored because I hadn't developed the education I needed, having skipped school in California.

It was during this period of my life that I actually discovered what dentistry was all about and decided that I wanted to become a dentist. I remember the event like it was yesterday. I was in eighth grade, and my cousin was getting married. He was in dental school, and he sat with me for about two hours. We talked about dentistry and about life in general. I saw how happy he was, and I wanted just a piece of what he had. I just wanted to experience the happiness he was experiencing.

After that talk, I knew I wanted to be a dentist, and I started making As and Bs. I went to high school at Enterprise High School in Alabama in the small town we moved to from California. It was a pretty cool high school, and I have a lot of fond memories there. When we first moved, it took a while to get into the "good old boy" network, but high school was fun and I had a good time. I made a lot of close friends.

After high school, I went to junior college for a year, and then on to the University of Alabama. My strategy was to go to a school that had a dental school. Even before I was accepted, I wanted to go to the dental school and learn as much as I could about dentistry. So I went to the University of Alabama, Birmingham, and majored in Biology and Chemistry. After graduation, I went straight into dental school.

To this day, I believe that dentistry saved my life, and I feel honored to be where I am right now in my life. I'm living beyond my wildest dreams.

Today, my partner, Jared Van Ittersum, and I own twelve dental practices in eight different states across the country. So when you look back at where I was and what has happened, it is almost unbelievable. I am now sur-rounded with incredibly talented and highly motivated people, and it's almost hard to take it all in. It's hard to feel like you deserve something like that.

Major Events That Shaped My Life

If you don't mind me getting a little philosophical here, we all have major events that shape our lives as we move forward. Besides the talk I had with my cousin that influenced me to turn my life around and become a dentist, there are several other factors that had an impact over the years.

One was the inability to be able to hang out with my father and to have a stable home life. That has really impacted my life, driving me to make sure that I provide a very stable home and life for my children. I remember one time my dad took me out fishing. I cherished that moment even then, and I remember similar moments with my father that I cherish today.

I always wanted to have a great family life, so I was willing to do whatever it took to get it. I think that's why dentistry has remained so attractive to me. Throughout the years, I've been able to set my own hours, have my own company, and be my own boss. It has always stuck with me that dentistry has limitless potential.

A part of Michigan influenced my life. I have an aunt and uncle, Lynn and Buck Boersma, who lived on Spring Lake in Michigan, and it was my heaven on earth growing up. It was the place that I would go to that was the life I always dreamed of. I remember we would sit out on the porch and Aunt Lynn would come out with some fresh fruit. Or we would be in the lake swimming, and when she came out, we would run up to the porch, eat, and then go back into the lake. We'd wake up in the morning, go out on the dock, look at the bass and the sun fish, and life was good. Why wouldn't it be, if all you have to do is fish, play in the water, run up to the house to eat, and then do it all over again?

Just being able to experience that life and see the relationship that my Aunt Lynn and my Uncle Buck had was incredible. They were high school sweethearts, and to this day, even after being married for thirty-six years, they still hug and kiss each other like they're in high school. By experiencing that life, I knew that it could be possible for anyone, including me. I knew that a strong marriage between two people who cared deeply for one another could be possible, and wanting that life really drove me to become a success. It was my dream life, the house on a lake with a beautiful wife and a wonderful family.

I now have a beautiful wife, Anne Claire, a beautiful nineteen-month-old daughter, Margot, and an awesome five-month-old son named after my dad, Elias. My wife comes from modest means; she was born and raised in a small house in a small town in Mississippi.

We're building our dream house in Nunica, MI as I'm writing this chapter. Having a stable home and growing up in one place is the one thing that I always wanted for my kids, as well as for myself.

Now I can provide that lifestyle for my children, and that really is very special for me.

Graduating from a dental school was also a major event in my life that has had a profound impact on me. To be quite honest, I never thought I was smart enough to even get into dental school, let alone get out of dental school. I think that while growing up, I didn't have the self confidence that a young adult should have. I just didn't feel like I could do it, and when I did graduate from dental school, it proved to me that I was smart enough and that I could accomplish my dreams and desires.

Another such event was getting accepted to the cross-country cycling team. That was the first time I ever got accepted to anything that I really wanted to do. This happened at a time when I was trying to get into dental school, and I had just been denied. When I got onto the team, I felt that I was finally part of something big. It allowed me to ride my bike across the United States with a team to benefit people with disabilities.

While I was on that cross-country ride, there was one moment that stands out in my memory and shows me that kindness can change someone's life. It was in California. We had stopped at a home for people with disabilities, and there was a lady with cerebral palsy who had been abandoned by her parents. This family found out about it, adopted her, and gave her a computer to communicate with. To this day, I remember walking up to her and putting my hand on her shoulder, and she smiled so big. I had never seen a smile this big before. She was smiling from ear to ear, and that's an under-statement. She had such a huge smile and I remember that moment touching me deeply. Even though we stopped every day at a home for people with disabilities, this one girl sticks out in my mind because all it took was a touch on her shoulder to make her happy.

That cross-country bike trip had a profound impact on me. It changed my perspective on life. It made me be thankful and appreciative of all the things we take for granted, such as just being able to walk, ride a bike, or take a deep breath and breathe naturally. From that moment with the girl, I learned that it isn't always the big things in life that leave lasting memories, but it can be something as simple as a touch on the shoulder, or simply giving someone an authentic smile.

I tell our dental team to show people that you're happy to see them and smile. You never know when a smile can change a life.

I remember the day I found out I was accepted to dental school. Most of the people had received their acceptance letters in December, and this was May. It was my third year of trying to get into dental school, and I hadn't heard anything one way or the other.

One day, I walked out of the house and went to the mailbox. There still wasn't a letter from the school in the box. At that time, literally everybody who applied was either getting a decline or an acceptance letter. So I called the admissions board at the school and asked, "I'm just wondering what's going on in my application?"

The girl on the other end of the phone replied, "Yeah, I think you were accepted. But let me check to make sure." And I remember my heart racing, like I felt that I was going to have a heart attack. Time stopped and I literally thought to myself, Oh my God, this is really happening. Is this really happening? Please come back and say that I really got accepted! She came back and said, "Yeah, I have the letter right here. We're gonna send this out. Yeah, you got accepted to dental school."

When I hung up the phone, I ran up and down the hall of the house I was renting. I was screaming and crying. I fell on my knees, and I was so excited that I sat there and prayed, literally, for an hour, just thanking God for getting me into dental school. I was so excited. I couldn't wait to tell everybody.

I called my dad and I said, "Dad, where are you?" He was driving, and I said, "Dad, you need to pull over." So he said okay and pulled over to the side of the road. I said, "Dad, I just got accepted into dental school!" and he screamed and cried. It was just an amazing event in my life and for my family, and the next week I got my acceptance letter from the University of Alabama. Later, the dean of admissions told me that "they had a little argument over who was going to call me because everybody was so excited to let me know that I was accepted into dental school, because they knew how hard I had tried to get in." I have to tell you, that was one of the best moments of my life.

Another huge event for me was meeting Gary Kadi. I had just purchased the practice in Whitehall, and I was lost. I didn't know anything about insurance, managing people, or anything else business related. All I knew about was practicing dentistry.

I have always battled with feeling like I deserve what I have. I had a very low deserve level and Gary Kadi was really able to coach me into becoming a stronger leader and believing in myself. I was able to learn some of his philosophies that helped me understand that life won't give you what you deserve, but what you feel you deserve.

Learning to have a healthy deserve level was a game changer for me, and I've since discovered that it's one of the pieces of the puzzle to achieve a successful life. In fact, I believe that it eventually led to Jared becoming my partner, and everything that has come from our partnership. It was like planting a seed, and from that one seed a whole garden would grow. Having Jared show up in my life was something that I never saw coming. Jared and I have come to discover how much we think alike, and we have become like brothers. From our relationship a whole garden of dental practices has grown.

My Philosophy About Dentistry

For you to understand how I care for my patients, it's important that you understand my philosophy about dentistry.

At first, I got into dentistry because you never have to sell anything. You get to set your own hours, and you get to make good money. Over time, my philosophy has changed. I've discovered that you have to make it all about your patients and your team because without a winning team, everybody loses. You lose. Your family loses at home because you're losing at work, and you bring that home with you. The patients lose because they aren't getting the treatment that they deserve. They deserve to be in a good environment right when they walk in; they deserve to hear laughter in the office.

So, my philosophy changed from centering around what kind of dentistry I want to do to focusing on what of kind of person I want to be. So it's not all about cosmetics or about technology. To me, it's all about how I can make my team happy, and in turn, how my patient is benefiting from the team being happy.

One of my beliefs is that you have to be able to change the lives of your team members so that they change the lives of the patients walking in the front door. You can have integrity as a doctor, but your patients don't know that. They learn about you by hearing what is being said in that exam room after you leave.

We can't expect excellent and energetic service to be routinely provided to our patients unless our team members (those with patient contact and those in support functions), who provide that exceptional service, are themselves engaged in an active personal pursuit of growth and excellence.

Our belief is that whether, they be doctors, hygienists, assistants, or front office team members, their purpose is to become the best version of themselves.

It's almost like the saying, "You build it and they will come." Well, if you build a positive environment, the patients will come, the money will come, the happiness will come, and you will be able to change the world through dentistry one patient at a time. That's my philosophy now.

Developing Something Better Than Corporate Dentistry

I know that there will be doctors who read this book and wonder how Infinity Dental Partners came about. So this is what happened.

My cousin had a satellite office-- in other words, a second office at a different location. So from early in my career, I started thinking: wouldn't it be nice to be able to have multiple locations, and what could happen if you have a group-type practice?

With a group practice, everybody could learn and benefit from each other. So I came out of school and had the idea that I wanted to have multiple practices. The problem was that dentistry had become so corporate, and when I was in dental school, everybody was talking about the issues with corporate dentistry. It was failing the patient miserably.

When Jared and I became partners and talked about our futures, I said, "Jared, wouldn't it be sweet if we could buy multiple practices but not make it 'corporate?'" And it was from those conversations with Jared that Infinity Dental Partners was born. We both felt the same way: we never wanted Infinity Dental Partners to be seen as "corporate dentistry."

We decided that in order to isolate ourselves from the image of corporate dentistry, we had to be invisible to the outside world. We felt that it was important to maintain the identity of the office that we were purchasing.

We decided that we didn't want to be simply one of the best of the best. We wanted to be the only ones who do what we do.

When we first started defining the idea of expanding our group practice, we wanted to create an environment in which everybody in the office had fun, from the team to the doctors. What we realized was that a lot of the doctors we talked to weren't having fun practicing dentistry anymore. The burden of having to manage the practice was exhausting and frustrating for many of them. We decided that, if we could eliminate the burden of management from the doctors so that they could focus on dentistry, it would remove a huge amount of stress from their lives and let them focus on what they loved to do.

We also knew that each dental office had its own DNA, and we didn't want to change that. We wanted to respect the practices' uniqueness; after all, in most practices the team has been together for years and developed their own way of doing things. So the challenge would be to manage the practice in a way that recognized this fact yet brought in systems that improved workflow, incorporated a higher level of patient education than most practices had ever seen, and made the office a fun place to work.

We wanted a group practice that would change people's lives for the better. So we started researching manage-ment companies and extracted the best parts of what each one was doing. Then we began implementing them into our practices to test each of the systems. If it didn't work as we anticipated that it would, we threw it out and kept only those parts that supported our goals. If it had a positive effect on our team members, our doctors, and our patients, we kept it and worked to improve it.

We developed Infinity Dental Partners into this group practice that is non-corporate and changes the lives of everybody associated with it. We are taking the best of everything we can find in dentistry, everything that has a positive impact on our teams', doctors', and patients' lives, and incorporating these systems, strategies, and philosophies into every office that becomes part of our organization. It works, and for Jared and me, it's been a truly humbling experience to see how we can impact so many lives in such a positive way.

I mentioned earlier in the chapter that Gary Kadi has had a big influence on me and my philosophy about dentistry, and here's why. Every year Gary Kadi invites about 15-20 doctors to a think tank about dentistry, and I was invited to go to Cancun, Mexico at the Ritz Carlton. For me it was a life-changing experience because we focused on where we wanted to take dentistry. In other words, we got to redefine ourselves as dentists and how we felt the industry should serve and care for its patients.

The topic the first day was: What is dentistry known as? It's stinky… It's smelly... It takes time out of the patient's day. It's not the "hip" medical profession. Being a dentist is not a "hip" thing to do. It's the profession with the highest suicide rate.

Then the second day, we talked about what we want to make dentistry known for. We wanted to be known as a profession that is changing lives. We wanted the profession to get the respect that it deserves. We wanted dentists to be educating patients on the mouth-to-body connection so that our patients could become healthier. We wanted to be the profession that is known to be very giving and life changing.

On the final day of this think tank, we had the responsibility of formulating a statement that would become our compass for how we wanted to move into the next era of dentistry. We came up with "pioneering total health and wellness for all."

Comprehensive Dentistry: "Pioneering Total Health And Wellness"

When you think of a pioneer, you think of a guy climbing over a mountain to get to the Promised Land. We're climbing this mountain of misconception of dentistry. In communities across the nation and in the medical field, people don't realize how connected the mouth is to the body. If we're going to change dentistry, we have to educate the public about this connection. After five years, this is beginning to happen, but there is still a lot of work to do.

If you picked up and are reading this book, I want to take a moment to provide you with some critical information you need to know.

There are endless studies showing how tooth loss leads to many years lost from your lifespan. There are studies showing the relationship of problems in your mouth to diabetes and low birth weight.

Knowing how the mouth is connected to the body, dentists can now catch problems in the operatory. Today we have the ability to take a pictographic image of your head and your neck, and in the digital image we can see the plaque that may be in your carotid arteries. We can educate you on what could happen if this is left untreated, and refer you to your cardiologist so that they can treat you. The bottom line is that there is a link between high quality of life and a healthy mouth.

Currently, Jared and I are talking about creating schools for health and wellness, where Infinity Dental Partner doctors can teach other doctors how to educate their patients effectively on total health. The goal is that the patient understands why a doctor is recommending a particular treatment plan and is motivated to accept treatment.

THE BENEFITS OF JOINING INFINITY DENTAL PARTNERS

I see Infinity Dental Partners as limitless. I fail to under-stand why a doctor wouldn't want to become part of Infinity Dental Partners. Currently, a doctor has to worry about the burden of management, wherein he is the CEO, the CFO, the marketing director, and the human relations manager. He is all these people, yet he says he wants to give the best care to his patients. We have found that a doctor performs his best when he is free of these responsibilities and can focus 100% on his patient.

A doctor has the responsibility of the operations, or the nuts and bolts of his practice, and he also has a responsi-bility to his patients. If you're so stressed out throughout the day about all the management stuff, how will your mind be 100% on that patient? What Infinity Dental Partners is doing for their doctors is taking the management burden off the doctor so they can focus on the patient.

So to me, it doesn't make sense not to become part of Infinity Dental Partners, where a dentist can become part of a movement to change dentistry and take it in the direction that it needs to go. That direction allows doctors to provide the highest level of patient care, keeping in mind the systemic relationship between the mouth and the body, to be able to focus 100% of your time on your patients and not have to deal with all the management issues. And finally, to become the best version of himself or herself because they interact with other doctors who are there to support their efforts and share their knowledge with one another.

Let me share what I believe is the biggest difference be-tween Infinity Dental Partners and what we know as the typical model of corporate dentistry: I would say it is our philosophy. Our philosophy is that if you change the lives of your team members, in turn you're going to change the lives of your patients. Furthermore, if you change the lives of the patients then you will change the world.

Corporate dentistry oftentimes will fire much of the staff who has been with a practice for a long time because their salaries tend to be higher than what they can hire a younger person for. We don't do that. We value older employees and understand that they have often built relationships with the patients in the practice. Why would we want to let go of someone who has a strong relationship, many times spanning decades, with a patient? Corporate dentistry is driven by the numbers and typically tells its doctors and hygienists that they have to hit certain numbers in order to keep their jobs. We don't do that either. We won't tell a doctor that he has to shorten the amount of time that he's going to be with his patients so that we can hit our goal that day. Our focus is one of providing the highest quality of dental care for our patients, educating them on how important it is to keep their mouths healthy, and retaining them as patients for their lifetimes.

We want everyone in our offices to connect with their patients and know what matters to each one individually. Patients are not just numbers to us; they are people who we know and see in the communities that we serve.

Furthermore, we don't come in and slap a sign on the front of your building that says "Infinity Dental Partners." We're not into mass marketing on TV. We are not into micromanaging by numbers. We believe in a philosophy of caring for our patients, our teams, and our doctors. If you believe in this philosophy, and you believe in a movement to change dentistry to a higher standard, everything will take care of itself. What we have found is that this belief has proven itself to hold true with all of our practices.

Making A Difference In People's Lives

One of the things that Jared and I believe is that it is important to find ways to give back to each of the communities we live in. One of the ways we found to do that is to hold a Free Dental Day.

The first Free Dental Day we ever held I will remember until the day I die. The day of the Free Dental Day, Jared and I were walking up to the office at five o'clock in the morning.

There was a line out of the parking lot. When I say line, I mean there were probably two hundred and fifty people lined up in the front of the building, and they were cheering us. They were clapping. They were just so excited that we were providing free dentistry to them because they simply couldn't afford it due to their life circumstances. We were so taken back because it was raining, and it was cold, and they'd been standing in line for hours. Some of them had been there since five o'clock the night before.

All we saw were smiles on their faces, showing just how happy everybody was to be there. We were so tired coming into the office at that hour, but by the time we walked through the front door we were stoked. You kind of get this adrenalin rush, and the team was excited too. The thrill of such an appreciative crowd of people was infectious.

I remember starting that day when this young girl walked in and sat in the chair. She must have been in her 20s or early 30s. She was noticeably shivering. We literally went out, got a blanket, and put it on her. We actually were worried about hypothermia because she had been sitting in this rain for so long. I noticed that she had a plastic bracelet on her wrist and I said, "That looks like a hospital bracelet. Did something happen?" She said, "Yes. I was in the hospital for a tooth infection, when somebody in the hospital told me that White Lake Family Dentistry is doing a free dental day. When I heard that, I checked myself out of the hospital without the permission of my physician. He said that I needed to stay there and get IV antibiotics." She said, "I know I need to see a dentist, but I didn't have any money to pay for the dentistry."

She was sitting there telling me this story with her eyes closed. Then I numbed her, and I could see her shoulders noticeably drop into the chair. Her whole body just went limp because that was the point I got her out of pain. I then removed the tooth, and she was crying. I was crying. Everybody was crying. Everybody was just very, very touched by the moment. And that's when I knew, right there, that the whole event was worth all the work that it took to make it happen.

That event told Jared and me that we had to do this every year in every one of our offices. Although it is just one of the ways we try to give back to the community, the fact is, we receive more than we ever gave to these people. We are all thankful that we are in a profession that lets us have such an impact on people's lives.

The Future of Dentistry

When I look at the direction in which dentistry is moving, it worries me. Without Infinity Dental Partners, I believe that dentistry is moving toward corporate dentistry, where it becomes about bonuses, and it becomes about how many people you can stuff into the chair during one day. It's about how many patients come through the front door. There's no doubt about it: that's the current path the profession is taking.

Jared and I have created Infinity Dental Partners to protect our profession from that ideology. The biggest difference is that we see corporate dentistry as dollar-driven, and Infinity Dental Partners' philosophy is patient-focused.

We want to consider the patients' personal motivators. What drives that patient to get up in the morning? If you don't know the most critical values of your patient, then you don't know your patient.

There is little doubt that dentistry is changing, and I believe that dentists are going to be on the front line of healthcare. It's almost to the point where the insurance companies are demanding an oral exam before a patient goes in for any type of surgery. We are beginning to see the public understand how important your mouth is to quality of life.

It's important to remember that almost everybody has teeth, and therefore, everybody needs a dentist. That gives dentists an opportunity to reach people and touch them in a way that can change their lives. We should never forget that. We should never forget how special dentistry is.

Like many dentists, I've been on a mission trip, and in the middle of a desert seen fifty people who have walked over a hundred miles to have a tooth removed. I've seen people line up two hundred and fifty deep to see us on our Free Dental Days. When you experience these events, you see just how important dentistry is to people all over the world, not just here in the United States. It drives home just how valuable our profession is.

(This content should be used for informational purposes only. It does not create a doctor-patient relationship with any reader and should not be construed as medical advice. If you need medical advice, please contact a doctor in your community who can assess the specifics of your situation.)

Printed in Dunstable, United Kingdom

91218906R00141